Marina Davila Ross

Towards the evolution of laughter

Marina Davila Ross

Towards the evolution of laughter

A comparative analysis on hominoids

Südwestdeutscher Verlag für Hochschulschriften

Impressum/Imprint (nur für Deutschland/ only for Germany)
Bibliografische Information der Deutschen Nationalbibliothek: Die Deutsche Nationalbibliothek verzeichnet diese Publikation in der Deutschen Nationalbibliografie; detaillierte bibliografische Daten sind im Internet über http://dnb.d-nb.de abrufbar.
Alle in diesem Buch genannten Marken und Produktnamen unterliegen warenzeichen-, marken- oder patentrechtlichem Schutz bzw. sind Warenzeichen oder eingetragene Warenzeichen der jeweiligen Inhaber. Die Wiedergabe von Marken, Produktnamen, Gebrauchsnamen, Handelsnamen, Warenbezeichnungen u.s.w. in diesem Werk berechtigt auch ohne besondere Kennzeichnung nicht zu der Annahme, dass solche Namen im Sinne der Warenzeichen- und Markenschutzgesetzgebung als frei zu betrachten wären und daher von jedermann benutzt werden dürften.

Verlag: Südwestdeutscher Verlag für Hochschulschriften Aktiengesellschaft & Co. KG
Dudweiler Landstr. 99, 66123 Saarbrücken, Deutschland
Telefon +49 681 37 20 271-1, Telefax +49 681 37 20 271-0, Email: info@svh-verlag.de
Zugl.: Hannover, TiHo and ZSN, Diss., 2007

Herstellung in Deutschland:
Schaltungsdienst Lange o.H.G., Berlin
Books on Demand GmbH, Norderstedt
Reha GmbH, Saarbrücken
Amazon Distribution GmbH, Leipzig
ISBN: 978-3-8381-0779-0

Imprint (only for USA, GB)
Bibliographic information published by the Deutsche Nationalbibliothek: The Deutsche Nationalbibliothek lists this publication in the Deutsche Nationalbibliografie; detailed bibliographic data are available in the Internet at http://dnb.d-nb.de.
Any brand names and product names mentioned in this book are subject to trademark, brand or patent protection and are trademarks or registered trademarks of their respective holders. The use of brand names, product names, common names, trade names, product descriptions etc. even without a particular marking in this works is in no way to be construed to mean that such names may be regarded as unrestricted in respect of trademark and brand protection legislation and could thus be used by anyone.

Publisher:
Südwestdeutscher Verlag für Hochschulschriften Aktiengesellschaft & Co. KG
Dudweiler Landstr. 99, 66123 Saarbrücken, Germany
Phone +49 681 37 20 271-1, Fax +49 681 37 20 271-0, Email: info@svh-verlag.de

Copyright © 2009 by the author and Südwestdeutscher Verlag für Hochschulschriften Aktiengesellschaft & Co. KG and licensors
All rights reserved. Saarbrücken 2009

Printed in the U.S.A.
Printed in the U.K. by (see last page)
ISBN: 978-3-8381-0779-0

TABLE OF CONTENTS

	Page
ABSTRACT	1
ZUSAMMENFASSUNG	2
GENERAL INTRODUCTION	4
CHAPTER 1: OCCURRENCE AND CONTEXT OF VOCAL LAUGHTER DURING SOCIAL PLAY IN ORANGUTANS	
Introduction	19
Methods	23
Results	31
Discussion	35
Acknowledgements	40
References	40
CHAPTER 2: RAPID FACIAL MIMICRY IN ORANGUTAN PLAY	
Introduction	43
Methods	44
Results	50
Discussion	52
Acknowledgements	54
References	55
CHAPTER 3: TOWARDS THE EVOLUTIONARY ORIGIN OF VOCAL LAUGHTER --- A COMPARATIVE ACOUSTIC AND PHYLOGENETIC ANALYSIS ON TICKLING VOCALIZATIONS OF GREAT APES AND HUMANS	
Introduction	58
Methods	60
Results	68
Discussion	75
Acknowledgements	80
References	80
GENERAL DISCUSSION	88
GENERAL ACKNOWLEDGEMENTS	98
GENERAL REFERENCES	100

ABSTRACT

A central question in evolutionary biology is to what extent humans share coding and decoding strategies of affective communication with great apes. Human laughter is of special interest for such comparative approach since it appears across all cultures and early in ontogeny and because its facial display shares commonalities with the nonhuman primate relaxed open-mouth (ROM) and open-mouth bared-teeth (OMBT) displays, which were also described as "laugh variants". Like in humans, these facial expressions of great apes may be accompanied by low-frequency (LF) vocalizations during tickling and social play.

In this thesis, we conducted a comparative analysis across hominoids (orangutans, gorillas, chimpanzees, bonobos, and humans) to assess the function, contagion, and evolution of their facial and vocal displays during tickling sessions and social play by using videographic and bioacoustic methods. Firstly, we assessed the function of LF vocalizations in orangutan social play and compared our results with those of previous studies on humans and chimpanzees. Our findings depicted partial support that LF play vocalizations activate playmates to continue with play and suggested phylogenetic continuity in this function for LF play vocalizations across hominoids. Secondly, we explored if orangutan open-mouth faces (e.g. ROM display and OMBT display) cause facial display congruency in conspecifics during social play. Results of this study showed that, similar to humans with laughter, orangutans mimic open-mouth faces of their playmates. Thirdly, we examined the acoustic properties and phylogeny of great ape LF vocalizations and human vocal laughter emitted when tickled using acoustic and phylogenetic analyses. Our findings revealed that these hominoid vocalizations showed the same topology as the one known from genetic studies. Therefore, we concluded that great ape LF vocalizations and human vocal laughter share the same phylogenetic origin and that the term vocal laughter is appropriate for these great ape vocalizations. Altogether, this thesis presented that laughter is not unique to humans, but that it emerged at least 12-16 million years ago.

ZUSAMMENFASSUNG

Eine zentrale Frage der Evolutionsbiologie ist, wie weit sich die Strategien der Kodierung und Dekodierung von affektiver Kommunikation bei Menschen und Großen Menschenaffen entsprechen. Das menschliche Lachen ist für solche Vergleiche von besonderem Interesse, da es in allen Kulturen und früh in der Ontogenie auftritt. Sein Gesichtsausdruck weist viele Gemeinsamkeiten mit dem relaxed open-mouth (ROM) display und dem open-mouth bared-teeth (OMBT) display von nichtmenschlichen Primaten auf, welche auch als "laugh variants" bezeichnet werden. Im Kontext des Kitzelns und sozialen Spiels können diese Gesichtsausdrücke bei Großen Menschenaffen, genauso wie beim Menschen, von low-frequency (LF) vocalizations begleitet sein.

Im Rahmen dieser These wurde eine vergleichende videographische und bioakustische Analyse von Gesichtsausdrücken und Vokalisationen von Hominoiden (Orang-Utans, Gorillas, Schimpansen, Bonobos und Menschen) beim Kitzeln und beim Spiel durchgeführt, um Fragen ihrer Funktion, Ansteckung und Evolution zu untersuchen. In der ersten Studie haben wir die Bedeutung von LF vocalizations im sozialen Spiel bei Orang-Utans erfasst und mit denen bisheriger Studien über Menschen und Schimpansen verglichen. Unsere Resultate wiesen darauf hin, dass LF vocalizations im Spiel die Spielpartner zum weiterspielen anregen und legten damit nahe, dass die Funktion dieser Vokalisationen bei den Homonoiden phylogenetisch kontinuierlich verläuft. In der zweiten Studie analysierten wir, ob das open-mouth face (u.a. ROM display und OMBT display) des Orang-Utans beim Spiel mit Artgenossen einen kongruenten Gesichtsausdruck hervorruft und dadurch ansteckend wirkt. Die Ergebnisse der Studie zeigten, dass Orang-Utans, ähnlich wie Menschen beim Lachen, das open–mouth face des Gegenübers imitieren. In der dritten Studie untersuchten wir mittels spezieller bioakustischer und phylogenetischer Verfahren die akustischen Eigenschaften und die Phylogenie von LF vocalizations bei Großen Menschenaffen und Menschen, die durch Kitzeln hervorgerufen werden. Der Stammbaum, der aufgrund der akustischen Eigenschaften von LF vocalizations erstellt wurde, weist dabei dieselbe Topologie auf, wie der aufgrund von genetischen Markern aufgestellte. Diese Studie belegt damit erstmals, daß nicht nur Menschen, sondern auch Große Menschenaffen, beim Kitzeln lachen können und daß das

Lachen des Menschen deshalb auf evolutionäre Wurzeln zurückzuführen ist, die mindestens 12-16 Millionen Jahre alt sind.

GENERAL INTRODUCTION

THE OBSCURITY OF HUMAN LAUGHTER

An integral question in neuroscience addresses humans' application of mental capacities as well as coding and decoding strategies in affective and referential communication. Human laughter is an important facial and vocal signal of affective and referential communication that has many unsolved puzzles. This makes a study on laughter's evolutionary root intriguing.

Although we mostly associate laughter with a socio-positive context (e.g. Grammer & Eibl-Eibesfeldt 1990), it also carries socio-negative functions (e.g. Blurton Jones 1967). Laughter is present with strong dependence on group composition (Provine 1993) and functions differently for either gender (e.g. Grammer & Eibl-Eibesfeldt 1990).

Laughter can also be self-rewarding (e.g. Mobbs et al. 2003), spontaneous or voluntary (e.g. Provine 2000; Wild et al. 2003), and contagious (e.g. Hatfield et al. 1994) and it can improve ones health and help lessen pain (Provine 2000) or be pathological (e.g. Ruch & Ekman 2001). It is often triggered by a surprise effect (e.g. van Hooff & Preuschoft 2003). And when heard too often, listeners may get annoyed (Provine 1992). Laughter occurs frequently in humor (e.g. Gervais & Wilson 2005) and casual conversation (e.g. Vettin & Todt 2004).

One way to evoke laughter is by tickling. However, there are also social factors influencing such evocation. Although we laugh when getting tickled by a person, that we know well and are fond of, such laughter does not occur when a stranger tickles us (e.g. Provine 2000).

Thus, laughter appears in many shapes and sizes that add to its complexity and nebulosity. In this study, human laughter was grasped at the roots of its functions, contagion, facial morphology and bioacoustics, socio-ecology, and evolution by assessing humans and our closest relatives, the great apes.

THE FUNCTION OF HUMAN LAUGHTER

The diversity of contexts in which human laughter appears makes it difficult to trace its functions. The most parsimonious and probably most informative approach to elucidate human laughter function is by studying the usage of children laughter and nonhuman primate play signals during social play or during tickling sessions. The following three hypotheses were proposed.

Laughter may function to activate others to continue with play (Rothbart 1973) (Play activation hypothesis, named by Matsusaka 2004). Furthermore, it is argued that rough play can quickly loose its playful side and escalate to real fights or other aversive behaviors (e.g. Bekoff 1999). To avoid such change in behaviors, playmates may signal a playful mood to playmates on the verge of becoming either fearful or angry (e.g. Caron 2002). This way, laughter of play could either be used to prevent an escalation in play by indicating a playful mood (Non-aggression hypothesis, named by Matsusaka 2004) or to protect oneself from getting injured by an angry playmate (Protection hypothesis, named in this study).

HUMAN LAUGHTER CONTAGION

One of the factors that add to the phenomenology of human laughter is its contagion. For the vocal (e.g. Smoski & Bachorowski 2003) and facial (e.g. Lundqvist 1995) manifestations of human laughter, findings indicated that people are prone to laugh while/after seeing or hearing laughter of another person. Besides yawning (e.g. Platek et al. 2003), smiling and laughter are probably the displays that trigger in humans most frequently congruent behaviors in every-day situations. Simply by mimicking happy faces, humans can perceive positive emotions (Lundqvist 1995). Thus, by means of display congruency, people may experience and understand the same emotions of others, a process that is termed emotional contagion (Hatfield et al. 1994). Emotional contagion most likely embodies an integral component of our social behavior.

FACIAL MORPHOLOGY OF HUMAN LAUGHTER

Zygomatic major (mouth corners back+up) and orbicularis oculi (eye wrinkles) are fundamental muscles that cause the typical facial manifestation of humans while laughing (reviewed in Ruch & Ekman 2001). Additionally, masseter and pterygoids are used for lowering the jaw. Gervais and Wilson (2005) distinguished between two displays of human laughter, namely Duchenne laughter and non-Duchenne laughter (see Figure 1). They argued that while the Duchenne laughter is driven by a stimulus and is an affective manifestation, the non-Duchenne laughter is self-generated and has no emotional meaning.

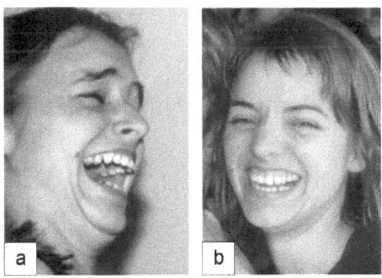

Fig. 1. Examples of facial expressions of an adult human while laughing. a) Duchenne laughter: driven by a stimulus and expressed in a positive emotional context of high arousal and b) non-Duchenne laughter: self-generated and emitted in context of no affective meaning.

BIOACOUSTIC CHARACTERIZATION OF HUMAN VOCAL LAUGHTER

Human vocal laughter can easily be recognized by others as laughter (e.g. Rothgänger et al. 1998). Although different syllables may be used in different cultures to express vocal laughter (Provine 2000), sound analyses showed that acoustic and temporal structures are much alike (e.g. Rothgänger et al. 1998).

However, vocal laughter also shows strong dynamics and a high level of diversity. For instance, Kipper and Todt (2001) found parametric dynamics of consecutive elements in rhythm and pitch rather than parametric consistency to make up "typical" laughter. Furthermore, laughter can consist of voiced (i.e. tonal) elements but also of unvoiced (i.e. atonal) elements with song-, grunt-, and snort-like expressions (Bachorowski et al. 2001). Interestingly, voiced laughter evokes more positive responses in listeners than unvoiced laughter (Bachorowski & Owren 2001; Grammer & Eibl-Eibesfeldt 1990). For three-year-old children, laughter was classified into the following (Nwokah et al. 1993): Exclamatory and dull comment; chuckle; basic, variable, and classical rhythmical; and squeal. Furthermore, there are individual (e.g. Rothgänger et al. 1998) and gender differences (e.g. Bachorowski et al. 2001) in its vocal production.

GREAT APE RELAXED OPEN-MOUTH AND OPEN-MOUTH BARED-TEETH DISPLAYS

In 1972, van Hooff proposed that the relaxed open-mouth (i.e. ROM) display (Figure 2), which often appears in nonhuman primate play and may be accompanied by staccato breathing (i.e. low-frequency play vocalizations), is the homologue of the human facial expression of laughter. The ROM display is an open-mouth expression, where the lower tooth row is bared (see Table 1 for morphological characteristics of ROM).

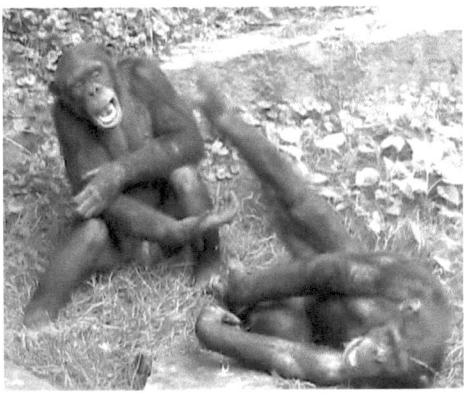

Fig. 2. ROM displays of two chimpanzees (9 and 10 years of age) during dyadic play.

Table 1. Overview of morphological characteristics and presence of staccato breathing (low-frequency play vocalization) for ROM display and OMBT display in accordance to Preuschoft (1995).

	Relaxed open-mouth display (i.e. ROM display)	Open-mouth bared-teeth display (i.e. OMBT display)
Lips	Loose or slightly retracted	Retracted
Teeth	Lower row bared, upper row covered	Bared
Mouth	Moderately to widely open	Wide open
Staccato breathing	Present	Present

Decades later, van Hooff and Preuschoft (2003) revised this view on laughter evolution by stating that nonhuman primates produce "laugh variants", which are open-mouth expressions ranging in the degree of baring the teeth. These authors argued that, in addition to the ROM display, an open-mouth display of showing no teeth and the relaxed open-mouth bared-teeth (i.e. OMBT) display belong to the category of "laugh variants" (i.e. open-mouth faces, in this study) (see Table 1 for morphological characteristics of OMBT). Similar to the ROM display, the OMBT display is produced in nonhuman primates during play (e.g. Preuschoft 1995) and can be accompanied by "panting laugh" (i.e. low-frequency play vocalizations) in great apes (e.g. de Waal 1988).

In their review, van Hooff and Preuschoft (2003) argued that the ROM display and OMBT display are both emitted by Old World monkeys, but that the former is more frequently produced by species phylogenetically more distanced to man, e.g. New World monkeys, prosimians, and canids, than the latter. This implies that the ROM display is ancestral to the OMBT display. Thus far, little is known about the occurrence of these two facial displays in great apes other than chimpanzees and bonobos. While the ROM display is more common in chimpanzees (e.g. Waller & Dunbar 2005), bonobos exhibit more frequently the full play face (i.e. OMBT display) (e.g. Palagi 2006). However, some chimpanzees may produce full play faces (i.e. OMBT displays) as frequently as they produce play faces (i.e. ROM displays) (Palagi 2006). Thus, these two displays may occur side by side within a species. They may also have different functions (e.g. Palagi 2006).

Besides occurring in the socio-positive context of play, the chimpanzee ROM display can be perceived by conspecifics as a positive state (Parr 2001), may reflect motivation to play (Waller & Dunbar 2005), and serve social bonding (Waller &

Dunbar 2005). To my knowledge, the OMBT display has not been investigated with these aspects.

Since smile and laughter are closely related in humans, nonhuman primates were also studied to shed light on the evolution of these manifestations. van Hooff (1972) argued that the phylogenetic precursor of smile is the nonhuman primate silent bared-teeth (SBT) display, which is exhibited in contexts of appeasement and affinity. He determined three distinct types of chimpanzee SBT displays, of which one, i.e. the "open-mouth SBT" display, showed morphological closeness to the human facial expression of laughter (Figure 3). Based on these morphological similarities of the "open-mouth SBT" display and based on findings that the ROM display can be accompanied by staccato vocalizations (low-frequency play vocalizations) during play, van Hooff (1972) proposed that the nonhuman primate SBT display converged morphologically with the ROM display to become laughter in humans (Emancipation hypothesis).

On the other hand, there are supporters of the Diminutive hypothesis (e.g. Redican 1982), who believe that smile and laughter both involve the same context, namely a "pleasant" one, and differ merely in their states of arousal. In accordance to this view, smile and laughter emerged from the same phylogenetic root.

GREAT APE LOW-FREQUENCY TICKLING/PLAY VOCALIZATIONS

Today, it is still uncertain whether vocal laughter evolved as an autapomorphy of humans or whether it originated on a prehuman basis. Numerous authors (e.g. Provine 2000; van Hooff 1972) agree that the most likely candidate for its nonhuman homologue is the great ape vocalization that can be evoked by tickling and also frequently occurs during social play. Due to their low-frequency ranges, I use the terms LF tickling vocalization and LF play vocalization, respectively, to describe these vocalizations (see Chapter 3, Figure 1 for spectrograms). Great ape staccato breathing (i.e. LF tickling/play vocalization) often accompanies ROM and OMBT displays (e.g. Chevalier-Skolnikoff 1982; Preuschoft 1995).

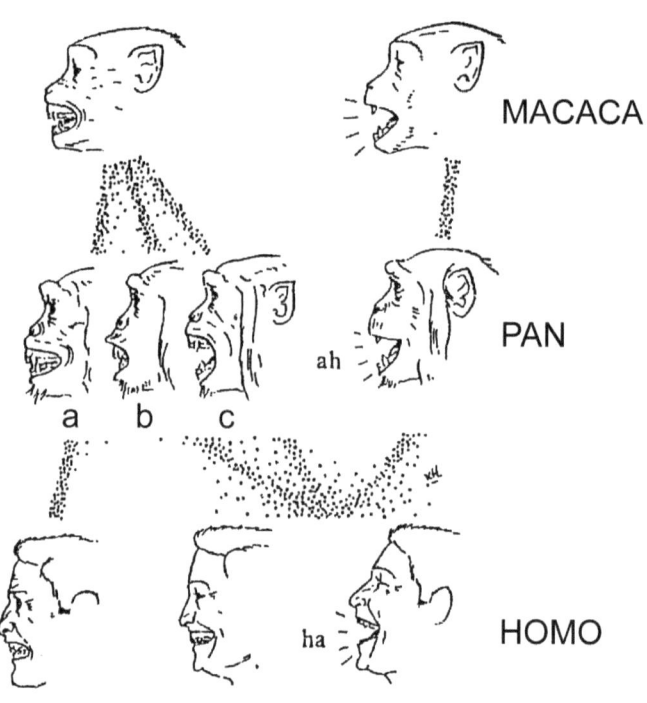

Fig. 3. Phylogenetic modifications of "smile" and "laughter" of macaques (*Macaca* spp.), chimpanzees (*Pan* spp.), and humans (*Homo* spp.) as suggested by van Hooff (1972). This graphic depicts smile and the SBT displays on the left side and laughter and the ROM display on the right side. The three chimpanzee SBT displays are a) horizontal SBT display, b) vertical SBT display, and c) open-mouth SBT display. In accordance to the Emancipation hypothesis, the open-mouth SBT display converged with the ROM display to ritualize as the facial expression of human laughter. Drawings were adapted from van Hooff (1972).

Thus far, only one study specifically assessed the function of great ape LF tickling/play vocalizations by testing the hypotheses on human laughter function (see above). In this study, Matsusaka (2004) showed that chimpanzees are more likely to continue with play after their playmates emitted play pantings (i.e. LF play vocalizations). This supported the Play activation hypothesis (see above). Furthermore, Matsusaka (2004) found no evidence that play pantings are used to signal "this is just play" to a playmate that may feel in danger of getting hurt and, thus, may stop playing. Consequently, Matsusaka (2004) rejected the Non-aggression hypothesis (see above).

While studying chimpanzees, Vettin and Todt (2005) argued that during rougher play, like wrestling, playmates cannot have much eye contact and, therefore, might be more likely to express play vocalizations than during less intensive play.

Thus far, all that is known about great ape LF tickling/play vocalizations is based on chimpanzees. These vocalizations of chimpanzees share acoustic commonalities with human vocal laughter in interval duration and intra- and interindividual variability (Vettin & Todt 2005).

However, while chimpanzees produce vocalizations with alternating exhalation and inhalation sounds during play and tickling (Vettin & Todt 2005), human vocal laughter is characterized by its series of consecutive expiratory sounds (Provine 1996). Provine (1996) suggested that limitations to modulate exhalation phases in chimpanzees, may be an integral factor of their incapability to speak besides, for instance, anatomic differences in the vocal apparatus (see Lieberman 1975).

To date, little is known about LF tickling/play vocalizations of great apes other than chimpanzees.

Comparative studies showed that orangutans, gorillas, chimpanzees, bonobos, and humans carry a rich vocal repertoire of tonal and atonal structures and can range from single calls (e.g. some screams) to long series of calls (e.g. long calls) (Table 2). Furthermore, Kojima (2001) found that auditory perception of pure tones was similar in human and chimpanzee infants.

Table 2: Comparative studies across hominoid vocal repertoires.

Study	Comment
Mitani 1996	Review of gorillas, chimpanzees, and bonobos in vocal behavior
Mori 1984	Comparison of chimpanzees and bonobos
Newman & Symmes 1982	Review of orangutan, gorilla, and chimpanzee infant vocalizations
Marler & Tenaza 1977	Review of orangutans, gorillas, and chimpanzees; facial manifestations associated to vocalizations
Marler 1976	Comparison of gorillas and chimpanzees
Ladygina-Kohts 1935/2002	Comparison of chimpanzee and human play, emotions, and vocal signals

SOCIO-ECOLOGICAL EFFECTS ON GREAT APE PLAY SIGNALS

It is important to note that socio-ecological factors may affect morphology, usage, and evolution of facial and vocal displays evoked during tickling and social play. Although these factors may be quite diverse across great apes, I roughly summarized their commonalities and differences as follows:

In orangutans (*Pongo* spp.), males live mostly solitary and females have individual overlapping home ranges (e.g. Delgado & van Schaik 2000; van Schaik 1999). Gorillas (*Gorilla* spp.) are more sociable than orangutans with groups of 3-21 members (Jenkins 1987). Chimpanzees (*Pan troglodytes*) and bonobos (*Pan paniscus*) live in fission-fusion communities of up to 100 and 200 individuals, respectively (reviewed in Rowe 1996). Of these two latter species, bonobos are more egalitarian (de Waal 1995, 2001). While orangutans and gorillas show a remarkable sexual dimorphism, this is less evident in *Pan*.

Preuschoft (1995) proposed the Power asymmetry hypothesis of motivational emancipation, in which species of despotic dominance systems produce more distinct displays of submission, affiliation, and playfulness than those of a more egalitarian social system. She argued that the articulateness of a signal, which could avoid fighting, may be more important for members of the former system. Her results on macaque SBT displays, ROM displays, and OMBT displays (as SBT-ROM intermediates) were compared to these displays of chimpanzees and human smile and laughter. Because these signals may occur differently across phylogenetically close species but may be used similarly in remotely related species, these authors predicted analogies. In tune with the argumentation of Preuschoft (1995), Palagi's (2006) study showed that the more egalitarian bonobos emit full play faces (i.e. OMBT displays) more often than the less egalitarian chimpanzees.

Furthermore, it was suggested that primates with less distinct sexual dimorphism may have less pronounced gender differences in play behavior than those with more apparent sexual dimorphism (Stevenson & Poole 1982).

TICKLING AND SOCIAL PLAY

Human listeners perceive great ape LF vocalizations of tickling as the same as those of social play (e.g. Chevalier-Skolnikoff 1982; Davila Ross, pers. obs.; Vettin & Todt 2005). Like in humans, tickling is also a component of great ape social play (siamangs: T. Geissmann pers. comm.; orangutans: Davila Ross pers. obs.; gorillas: e.g. Fossey 1972; e.g. chimpanzees: Matsusaka 2004; e.g. bonobos: de Waal 1988).

However, thus far, it is not known if tickling and social play contexts are homologous. Since the chapters of this thesis focused on displays of tickling sessions and social play, I aimed to clarify the phylogenetic relationship between these two sound-releasing contexts as presented in Table 3.

Table 3. The relative frequency of four facial displays in orangutans (N=10) while emitting LF vocalizations (n=218) during tickling sessions (n=97) with human ticklers. Tickling sessions were conducted according to Chapter 3. Tickling sessions were video-recorded and the presence of LF tickling vocalizations and four facial displays (open-mouth face, bite face, relaxed face, and nonrelaxed face) were coded in accordance to Chapters 1 and 2, respectively. The number of vocal events was scored for each facial display per orangutan. Each number of the respective facial display was divided by their total number per individual and multiplied by 100. Thereafter, means, standard deviations, and ranges of the four facial displays, respectively, were calculated for all orangutans.

Individual identification	Open-mouth face	Bite face	Relaxed face	Nonrelaxed face
1	50	0	0	50
2	63	0	0	37
3	50	25	0	25
4	69	31	0	0
5	97	0	0	3
6	86	0	0	14
7	32	0	0	68
8	77	8	0	15
9	55	15	0	30
10	59	0	0	41
Mean	63.8	7.9	0	28.3
Standard deviation	19.1	11.8	0	21.4
Range	32-97	0-31	0-0	0-68

Table 3 shows the relative frequency of four facial displays of orangutans (open-mouth face, bite face, nonrelaxed face, and relaxed face) while emitting LF vocalizations during tickling sessions with human ticklers. These facial displays were selected as they appear in orangutan social play (Davila Ross pers. obs.; also see Chapter 2, Table 1 for definitions).

Our results showed that orangutans mostly exhibited open-mouth faces (64%) (i.e. ROM and OMBT displays) (Figure 4) and nonrelaxed faces (29%) while emitting LF tickling vocalizations. These vocalizations were also displayed together with bite faces. However, since ticklers regularly avoided getting bitten by the orangutans, values on bite faces are expected to be higher than shown (8%). LF tickling vocalizations were never produced together with relaxed faces.

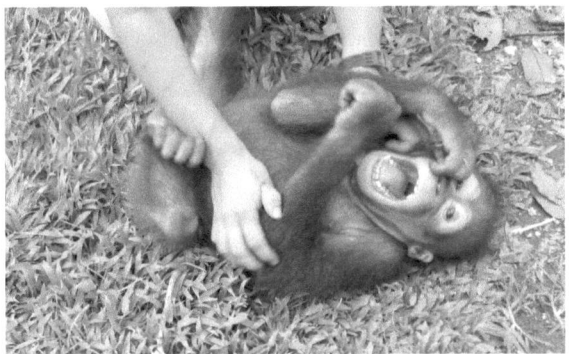

Fig. 4. Open-mouth face of a male orangutan (3 years of age) when tickled by a familiar human.

Orangutans also presented the same facial displays (open-mouth faces, bite faces, nonrelaxed faces) while producing LF vocalizations during social play (Davila Ross unpubl. data). Thus, I consider tickling sessions and social play with conspecifics as homologous sound-releasing contexts.

AIMS OF THIS STUDY

Using videographic and bioacoustic methods, I studied great ape open-mouth faces (e.g. ROM and OMBT displays) as well as great ape LF tickling/play vocalizations and human laughter in their function (Chapter 1), contagion (Chapter 2), and evolution (Chapter 3).

Chapter 1

Since our knowledge on the function of great ape LF play vocalizations is solely limited to chimpanzees (e.g. Matsusaka 2004), I assessed LF vocalizations of orangutan play in order to shed light on this topic while leaning on the three hypotheses on human laughter. 1) Play activation hypothesis: Orangutan LF play vocalizations activate playmates to continue with play (Rothbart 1973). 2) Non-aggression hypothesis: Orangutan LF play vocalizations indicate a playful mood and prevent playmates from discontinuing play out of fear from getting hurt (Caron 2002). 3) Protection hypothesis: Orangutan LF play vocalizations indicate a playful mood and protect callers themselves from getting injured by an angry playmate (Caron 2002). A similar study on chimpanzees showed support for the Play activation hypothesis (Matsusaka 2004).

Chapter 2

Preston and de Waal (2002) postulated phylogenetic continuity of empathic components between animals and humans as they facilitate social species by forming and keeping social bonds. Although display congruency is an integral component that adds to the phenomenology of human laughter, thus far, it was not assessed if it is present for the proposed homologous nonhuman primate modes of the human Duchenne laughter. Based on the commonalities between nonhuman primate open-mouth faces (e.g. ROM and OMBT displays) and the human Duchenne laughter (see above), I hypothesized that open-mouth faces can trigger facial congruency in orangutans during social play. In this study, I specifically assessed rapid (within 1 second) facial responses.

Chapter 3

Since human laughter is a cross-cultural phenomenon (e.g. Ekman 1973) and is emitted by infants from the age of four months onwards (e.g. Scheiner et al. 2002), newborns with gelastic epilepsy (Ruch & Ekman 2001), and deaf-blind children (e.g. Eibl-Eibesfeldt 1985), I postulated that human vocal laughter has a prehuman basis. Because of the many commonalities between great ape LF tickling/play vocalizations and human vocal laughter (see above), I phylogenetically analyzed LF tickling vocalizations of orangutans, gorillas, chimpanzees, and bonobos and human vocal laughter. Hereby, I predicted that these vocalizations share the same phylogenetic root. A resulting tree of these vocalizations that coincides with the widely accepted systematic topology of hominoids based on genetic studies (e.g. McBrearty & Jablongski 2005; Ruvolo et al. 1994; Wildman et al. 2002) (Figure 5), would confirm such homology.

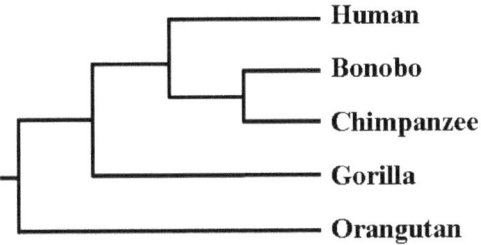

Fig. 5. Systematics of great apes and humans based on genetic studies (e.g. McBrearty & Jablongski 2005; Ruvolo et al. 1994; Wildman et al. 2002).

CHAPTER 1

OCCURRENCE AND CONTEXT OF VOCAL LAUGHTER DURING SOCIAL PLAY IN ORANGUTANS

INTRODUCTION

The evolution of human vocal laughter is still a mystery. Particularly the many functions and characteristics of human laughter make it difficult to understand how its vocal display emerged. Although we mostly associate human laughter with joy (e.g. Grammer & Eibl-Eibesfeldt 1990), it also can be aggressive (e.g. Blurton Jones 1967) and appeasing (e.g. Rothgänger et al. 1998). Furthermore, human laughter can be self-rewarding (Provine 2000), cognitively linked (e.g. Weisfield 1993) but also spontaneous (e.g. Dimberg & Thunberg 1998), and contagious (e.g. Provine 1992). It may also involve high arousal (e.g. Rothbart 1973), discomfort (e.g. Harris 1999), and surprise (e.g. Sroufe & Wunsch 1972).

From human studies, three main hypotheses on the function of laughter in play, that could depict its evolutionary origin, have been put forth. Laughter can be an expression of high arousal that activates the laughers' playmates to initiate or continue with play (Play activation hypothesis, named by Matsusaka 2004) (e.g. Harris 1999; Rothbart 1979). Based on evidence that rough play can escalate into real fights and/or can cause a playmate to get injured (e.g. Bekoff 1999), the following postulations were stated. By laughing, laughers can signal their playful moods to a fearful playmate (Non-aggression hypothesis, named by Matsusaka

2004) and/or to an aggressive playmate (<u>Protection hypothesis</u>, named in this study) (e.g. Caron 2002).

To elucidate how human vocal laughter evolved, it is essential to assess our closest relatives, the great apes. Human vocal laughter and great ape low-frequency (LF) vocalizations, that are evoked when tickled by humans, share the same phylogenetic origin (see Chapter 3). These tickling vocalizations (i.e. vocal laughter) of great apes are perceived by human listeners as the same as LF vocalizations of great ape social play (e.g. Davila Ross pers. obs.; Vettin & Todt 2005), which also can include tickling components (e.g. Fossey 1983; Goodall 1986). When vocally laughing during tickling sessions, orangutans displayed open-mouth faces, bite faces, and nonrelaxed faces (see General Introduction, Table 3; also see Chapter 2, Table 1 for definitions). The former facial display included an open-mouth expression of baring no teeth, the relaxed open-mouth (ROM) display, and the relaxed open-mouth bared-teeth (i.e. open-mouth bared-teeth or OMBT) display, which were proposed as "laugh variants" by van Hooff & Preuschoft (2003) (also see General Introduction, Table 1 for morphological characteristics). Since orangutans also show open-mouth faces, bite faces, and nonrelaxed faces while producing LF vocalizations during social play (Davila Ross pers. obs.), the term vocal laughter in this study covers LF vocalizations of tickling sessions with humans and those of play with conspecifics.

Thus far, our knowledge on the function of great ape vocal laughter is based on two chimpanzee studies. Using playback tests, Berntson et al. (1989) showed that infant chimpanzees responded to laughter with threat-like behavior, i.e. cardiac acceleration and vocalizations reminiscent of adult threat-barks. Interestingly, Berntson et al.'s (1989) finding contradicted all three laughter hypotheses. However, infant subjects were hand-reared and lived in peer-groups. Thus, their rearing history combined with the fact the caller was an unknown older chimpanzee may explain these results.

In his study on chimpanzee social play, Matsusaka's (2004) explicitly tested the Play activation and Non-aggression hypotheses. Firstly, he demonstrated that chimpanzees more likely maintained their play actions when their playmates emitted play pantings (i.e. vocal laughter). The author interpreted this result in that play pantings are expressions of high arousal/thrill and can activate the other playmates to continue with play. This supports the Play activation hypothesis. Notably, Matsusaka (2004) found that chimpanzees did not play pant to initiate play.

Secondly, Matsusaka (2004) identified laughers of "aggressive" play, which was described as an action that may also appear during aggression and predation (e.g. mouthing, chase, and slap). He found that targets of "aggressive" play were play panting more often than performers of "aggressive" play, especially when the former were infants and the latter were adolescents/adults. To infants, play with older playmates should involve a higher risk of getting injured than play with peers. Therefore, if older playmates would have emitted play pantings more often when playing with younger playmates, this should have indicated that play pantings are used to lessen the ambiguity of dangerous play to a playmate that could otherwise stop to play out of fear. Based on these grounds, Matsusaka (2004) rejected the Non-aggression hypothesis. Notably, Matsusaka's (2004) results could also be explained by the Protection hypothesis. See Table 1 for an overview of Matsusaka's (2004) findings with respect to the three laughter hypotheses.

So far, the function of vocal laughter in great apes other than chimpanzees (Berntson et al 1989; Matsusaka 2004) was not assessed in any study. Since orangutans represent the great ape species phylogenetically most distanced to humans and chimpanzees (e.g. Ruvolo et al. 1994), such study on orangutans could lucidify phylogenetic continuity or discontinuity of vocal laughter function across hominoids. Thus, for a better understanding on the evolution of hominoid vocal laughter function, it is of special importance to study orangutans.

Table 1. Overview of findings on functions of chimpanzee play pantings (i.e. vocal laughter) by Matsusaka (2004) and statements on support or rejection of the three main laughter hypotheses.

	Play activation hyp.	Non-aggression hyp.	Protection hyp.
• Individuals more likely continued to play after their playmates emitted play pantings (i.e. vocal laughter).	Yes	-	-
• Targets of "aggressive" play emitted play pantings most often.	-	No	Yes
• Infant targets of "aggressive" play were play panting more often during play with adolescents/adults.	-	No	Yes

No=Rejects hypothesis
Yes=Supports hypothesis
-=Not applicable for testing hypothesis

In this study, we investigated how vocal laughter functions in orangutan social play. Leaning on Matsusaka's (2004) chimpanzee study and on human studies (see above), the following hypotheses were tested for orangutan vocal laughter:

- Hyp. 1: The Play activation hypothesis suggests that laughter is produced to initiate play and/or to maintain play. If vocal laughter is an expression of high arousal/thrill and activates others to play, then laughers and their playmates (i.e. nonlaughers) should both prolong their play once vocal laughter is emitted. Furthermore, vocal laughter should occur shortly prior to play.

- Hyp. 2: The Non-aggression and Protection hypothesis implies that laughter is used to signal playfulness to fearful and aggressive playmates, respectively. It is most likely that younger playmates are at higher risk of getting injured during play than older playmates. Thus, if older playmates emit vocal laughter more frequently, this would imply that vocal laughter lessens the ambiguity of dangerous play by signaling to the younger playmate that there is no danger of an escalation into aggression. Such signaling behavior could, then, prevent that the younger playmate stops to play out of fear of getting hurt. Alternatively, if younger playmates laughed more often, it would suggest that vocal laughter is used to protect laughers themselves from getting hurt.

METHODS

Data collection, definitions, and videometric analyses

Orangutan dyadic play was video-recorded at Sepilok Orangutan Rehabilitation Centre (SORC), Malaysia, from August to October 2005. Observation times were between 8 a.m. and 12 a.m. and between 2 p.m. and 6 p.m.

SORC orangutans lived in two separate groups that represented individuals of different age classes and of different phases of the rehabilitation process. The Outdoor nursery consisted of orangutans >4 years of age that lived in a forest area of

2 km^2 and were free to enter the Sepilok Forest Reserve. Data on Outdoor nursery orangutans were collected at two feeding platforms within this forest area. The Indoor nursery included orangutans ≤5 years of age that were housed with peers. To record data on Indoor nursery orangutans, 2-5 subjects of similar age were taken outside to play.

A total of 322 orangutan dyadic play bouts of 64 playmate constellations (i.e. dyads) were collected ad libitum from 13 Indoor orangutans (40 dyads) and 8 Outdoor orangutans (24 dyads) using continuous recordings (see Table 2). Since orangutans had different histories and some individuals most likely were socially deprived prior to coming to SORC, subjects of this study were only orangutans that were observed to play with more than one playmate, independent of whether or not their play was video-recorded. Good-quality recordings were selected from <6 meters away from subjects. This reduced the number of play bouts to 302, while the number of dyads (N=64) and subjects (N=21) remained unchanged. See Table 2 for information on subject age, gender, age at SORC-admittance, total dyadic play duration, and recorder. Age groups were defined after Watts and Pusey (1993): Infants (0-4 years of age), juveniles (4-9 years of age), and subadults (9-12 years of age).

In accordance to Fagen (1981), play consists out of variable, repeated, and/or recombined functional behaviors outside their main contexts. All duration and frequency values were videometrically analyzed using a resolution of 3-4 frames with Interact 7.25 (Mangold, Arnstorf, Germany). Dyadic play bout durations started from the first frame where one playmate responded to the play invitation of the other playmate and ended when at least one playmate was not participating in play anymore for ≥500 frames (i.e. ≥20 seconds) or at the first frame when a third individual interfered. Nonplay phases of <500 frames (i.e. <20 seconds) between play bouts were termed as play breaks.

Table 2. Studied subjects of Indoor and Outdoor nursery at Sepilok Orangutan Rehabilitation Centre (SORC) with subject identification number and information on age, gender, age of admittance to SORC, total dyadic play duration, and recorder. Subjects that emitted vocal laughter are indicated in bold.

Group	Indiv. ID[1]	Age in months	Age in years	Gender	Age at SORC-admittance (in years)	Total dyadic play duration (in seconds)	Recorder[1]
Indoor nursery	I1	16	1.3	Male	1.0	77.64	MDR
	I2	21	1.8	Female	1.0	120.0	MDR
	I3	32	2.7	Female	2.0	700.50	MDR
	I4	**33**	**2.8**	**Male**	**1.0**	**1370.42**	**MDR**
	I5	34	2.8	Female	0.1	265.22	MDR
	I6	36	3.0	Female	1.0	568.00	MDR
	I7	38	3.2	Male	1.0	854.34	MDR
	I8	42	3.5	Female	2.0	160.68	MDR
	I9	**42**	**3.5**	**Female**	**0.8**	**772.02**	**MDR**
	I10	**43**	**3.6**	**Male**	**2.0**	**1700.62**	**MDR**
	I11	45	3.8	Male	1.0	512.22	MDR
	J1	61	5.1	Female	1.0	271.04	MDR
	J2	65	5.4	Female	2.0	482.42	MDR
Outdoor nursery	J3	57	4.8	Male	1.0	2625.82	MW
	J4	66	5.5	Male	1.5	3659.76	MW
	J5	**72**	**6.0**	**Male**	**1.0**	**3827.06**	**MW**
	J6	**84**	**7.0**	**Male**	**1.0**	**4593.40**	**MW**
	J7	**85**	**7.1**	**Male**	**5.0**	**5008.70**	**MW**
	J8	**105**	**8.7**	**Male**	**1.0**	**3178.90**	**MW**
	J9	106	8.8	Male	1.0	1720.70	MW
	S1	**145**	**12.1**	**Male**	**1.5**	**4518.38**	**MW**

[1] Abbreviations: I = infant; Indiv. ID = individual identification; J = juvenile; MDR = Marina Davila Ross; MW = Miriam Wessels; No. = number; S = subadults

Furthermore, the presence of vocalizations, play contexts, and play intensities were videometrically coded for each playmate separately. Vocalizations during play were defined as vocal laughter and play squeaks (see Chapter 3, Figure 1 for spectrogram). Eight play contexts were scored either as play of physical contact with slow grappling, tickling, fast grappling, gnawing, wrestling, hitting, and jumping or as play of no physical contact, e.g. play chase or when at least one playmate was slapping hands on the ground while sitting opposite the other (see Table 3 for definitions of play contexts). Since data were coded on an individual level, both playmates could concurrently display different play contexts, respectively. For play intensity, the seven play contexts of physical contact were grouped after Flack et al. (2004) into low (slow grappling/tickling), mid (fast grappling/gnawing/wrestling), and high (hitting/jumping) play intensity (see Table 3).

Videos were analyzed by one main observer. Inter-observer reliability was tested by the main and a second observer with one-frame accuracy. Cohen's Kappa mean agreements of 0.84 for the presence of vocalizations (20 bouts) and 0.89 for play contexts (21 play bouts) were excellent (Fleiss et al. 2003).

Medians were calculated if data values were ≤5. Means were calculated if values were >5.

Of the 302 analyzed play bouts (64 dyads), a total of 54 vocal laughter events were found in 13 play bouts for 10 dyads. For 42 vocal laughter events, laughers (N=9) could be identified in 12 play bouts for 9 dyads (n=10 nonlaughers). For 40 of these 42 vocal laughter events, play contexts/intensities could be identified at the onset of these events (N=9 laughers, n=9 dyads, n=12 play bouts). These vocal laughter events overlapped in their durations with 51 play contexts. See Table 2 for laugher and nonlaugher identification and Tables 4 & 5 for distribution of play bout occurrences per dyad with and without vocal laughter.

Table 3. Definitions and pictorial examples of the eight play contexts and their categorization to play intensities.

Play context*	Play intensity**	Definition	Example
Slow grappling	Low	At least one playmate held the other with hands/feet and moved slowly and relaxed.	
Tickling	Low	One playmate held the other playmate with hands/feet and pocked with moving fingers the other playmate's body.	
Fast Grappling	Mid	At least one playmate held the other with hands/feet and moved quickly and abruptly.	
Gnawing	Mid	At least one playmate slowly and continuously chewed on some body part of the other playmate.	
Wrestling	Mid	Playmates were rough and tumbling while in close bodily contact with each other.	
Hitting	High	One playmate was audibly slapping body part of other playmate.	
Jumping	High	One playmate suddenly bounced off/on the other playmate.	
Play of no physical contact		Playmates had no physical contact to one another, e.g. play chase or when at least one playmate was slapping hands on the ground while sitting opposite the other.	

*= in accordance to Flack et al. (2004) and Vettin and Todt (2005)
**= in accordance to Flack et al. (2004)

Table 4. Distribution of play bout occurrences per dyad of Indoor nursery orangutans (n=40 dyads; n=194 play bouts). Dyads with vocal laughter are indicated in bold. Numbers of play bouts with vocal laughter are depicted in brackets. Since Indoor nursery orangutans lived in peer enclosures and were taken out to play in groups of 2-5 as peers with small age differences or as peers that stayed together outside, not all 78 play dyads were theoretically possible.

	I1	I2	I3	I4	I5	I6	I7	I8	I9	I10	I11	J1	J2
I1	-	-	-	-	-	-	-	-	-	-	-	-	-
I2	0	-	-	-	-	-	-	-	-	-	-	-	-
I3	0	1	-	-	-	-	-	-	-	-	-	-	-
I4	0	0	15	-	-	-	-	-	-	-	-	-	-
I5	2	0	11	8	-	-	-	-	-	-	-	-	-
I6	0	0	3	2	1	-	-	-	-	-	-	-	-
I7	1	0	14	6	2	10	-	-	-	-	-	-	-
I8	0	0	0	0	0	2	0	-	-	-	-	-	-
I9	0	0	2	**9[1]**	1	0	0	0	-	-	-	-	-
I10	0	0	14	**5[2]**	1	6	**11[3]**	1	6	-	-	-	-
I11	0	0	10	0	1	11	1	1	4	4	-	-	-
J1	0	0	0	2	0	4	0	0	1	**3[1]**	0	-	-
J2	0	0	0	3	0	2	0	2	1	0	10	0	-

Occurrence of vocal laughter in orangutan social play

To calculate the percentage of vocal laughter across all play bouts of a dyad (N=64 dyads, n=302 play bouts), the number of play bouts with vocal laughter (n=13) was divided by the total number of play bouts and multiplied by 100. Then, its mean percentage was calculated across all dyads.

In order to obtain play bout durations with and without vocal laughter for each dyad (N=10 dyads, n=13 play bouts), mean/median durations of all play bouts with vocal laughter and of all play bouts without vocal laughter, respectively, were calculated per dyad. On the dyad level, play bout durations with vocal laughter were compared to play bout durations without vocal laughter using the Wilcoxon test.

Table 5. Distribution of play bout occurrences per dyad of Outdoor nursery orangutans (n=24 dyads; n=108 play bouts). Dyads with vocal laughter are indicated in bold. Numbers of play bouts with vocal laughter are depicted in brackets. Since Outdoor nursery orangutans were moved freely in the forest, 28 play dyads were theoretically equally often possible.

	J3	J4	J5	J6	J7	J8	J9	S1
J3	–	–	–	–	–	–	–	–
J4	8	–	–	–	–	–	–	–
J5	8	6[1]	–	–	–	–	–	–
J6	7	8	8	–	–	–	–	–
J7	3	4	5[1]	0	–	–	–	–
J8	3	1	5	7[1]	0	–	–	–
J9	0	2	2	1	0	2	–	–
S1	2[1]	1	3	6[1]	5	8[1]	3	–

Furthermore, the percentages of vocal laughter occurrences during the eight play contexts and play break was assessed. At each first frame where vocal laughter (n=40) occurred, the type of play contexts+break was scored. The total number of respective play contexts+break categories was counted for each dyad of every laugher (N=9 laughers, n=12 play bouts). To calculate the percentage of the respective play contexts+break category for every dyad, each value per dyad was divided by their total number of the respective dyad and multiplied by 100. Then, the mean percentages were calculated across all dyads for each laugher.

We also assessed vocal laughter durations of the three respective play intensities. For every dyad with vocal laughter (N=9), the durations of vocal laughter events (n=40) of the respective play intensity that occurred at the onset of the vocal laughter events were summarized per laugher. Afterwards, median durations were calculated for all dyads per laugher.

Characterization of laughers and nonlaughers

To test Hypothesis 1, play context continuity of laughers and nonlaughers was assessed. For every laugher (N=9), durations of play contexts (n=51 play contexts) were measured for each of the eight play contexts, respectively. Mean/median durations of the respective play contexts were calculated for each play bout per dyad per laugher, then for all play bouts per dyad per laugher, and finally for all dyads per laugher. The same procedure as above for play context durations with vocal laughter was carried out for play context durations without vocal laughter (n=48 play contexts) for the same dyads and individuals. On an individual level, the mean/median play context durations with vocal laughter were compared to the mean/median play context durations without vocal laughter using the Wilcoxon test.

For every nonlaugher (N= 10), the same calculations as above for the laugher were conducted (n=51 play contexts with vocal laughter).

Play initiation

To assess if vocal laughter is used to initiate play, the number of vocal laughter events that occurred 125 frames (i.e. 5 seconds) prior to the play bout onsets was scored. Furthermore, the number of vocal laughter events that occurred 125 frames (i.e. 5 seconds) after the play bout onsets was scored.

Characterization of younger and older playmates

To test Hypothesis 2, laughers were characterized depending on their playmate status (i.e. younger/older than the other playmate). The frequencies of all vocal laughter events were scored for the respective playmate status for each play bout per dyad per laugher (N=9 laughers, n=12 play bouts). Then, the medians of the respective playmate status were calculated for all play bouts per dyad per laugher. Afterwards, the medians of the respective playmate status were assessed for all dyads per laugher. Finally, the mean frequencies of vocal laughter between younger and older playmates were compared on an individual level using the Binomial test.

RESULTS

Occurrence of vocal laughter in orangutan social play

Vocal laughter occurred in 3.8% of all play bouts.

Table 2 depicts that 3 of 10 infants, 5 of 9 juveniles, and 1 of 1 subadult vocally laughed. Since some individuals played in more than one dyad where vocal laughter was emitted, our data revealed a discrepancy with 9 laughers and 10 nonlaughers.

For dyads where vocal laughter occurred, play bout durations with vocal laughter were significantly longer than play bout durations without vocal laughter (Wilcoxon matched-pairs signed-ranks: $Z=2.429$; N=10 dyads; $p=0.015$) (Figure 1).

Figure 2 shows the percentages of vocal laughter occurrences for each of the eight play contexts and play break per dyad with vocal laughter per laugher (N=9). Most orangutans (N=6) vocally laughed during wrestling. Vocal laughter was also present during slow grappling, fast grappling, gnawing, and play break, but absent during tickling, hitting, jumping, and play of no physical contact.

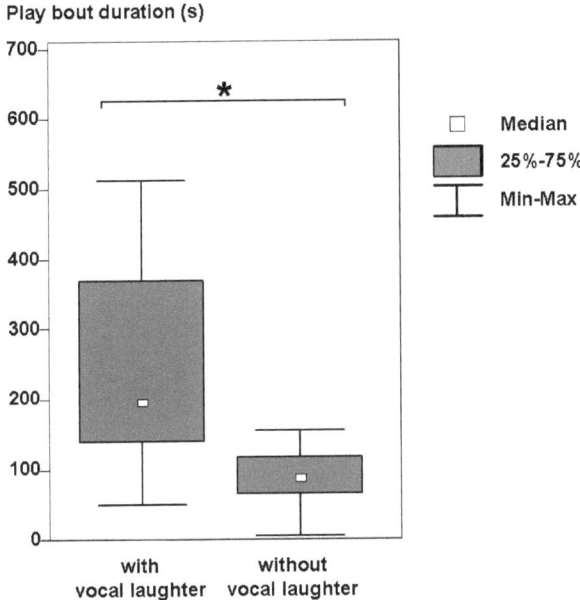

Fig. 1. Play bout duration with vocal laughter and without vocal laughter per dyad (N=10). Bouts with vocal laughter were significantly longer (Wilcoxon matched-pairs signed-ranks: Z=2.429; p=0.015).

Figure 3 depicts vocal laughter durations for each of the three play intensities per dyad per laugher. Vocal laughter was present during low and mid play intensity, but absent during high play intensity.

Duration of play contexts in relation to vocal laughter: Laughers versus nonlaughers

For Hypothesis 1, the play context duration with and without own vocal laughter was assessed for laughers (Figure 4). The play contexts lasted significantly longer when vocal laughter occurred (Wilcoxon matched-pairs signed-ranks: Z=1.955; N=9 orangutans; p=0.050). Notably, its p-value borders at the threshold of significance.

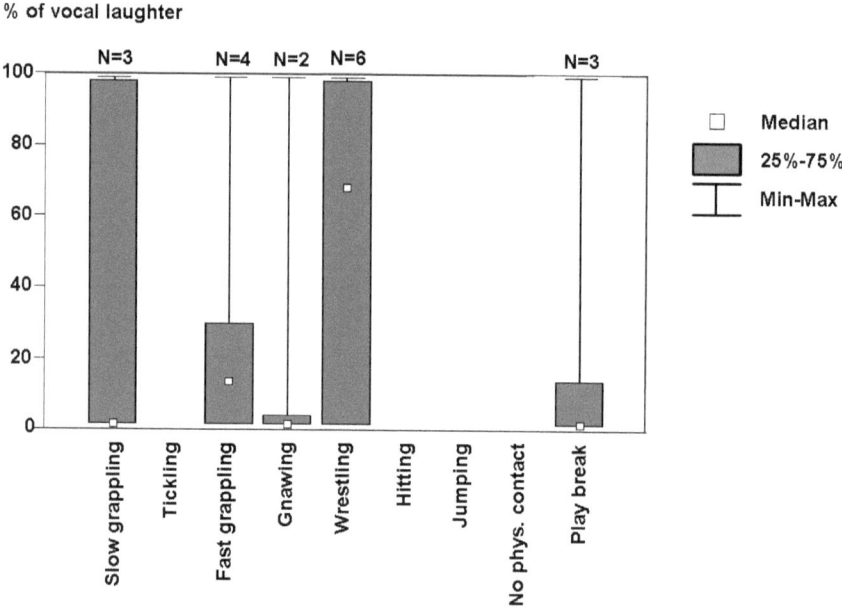

Fig. 2. Percentage of vocal laughter occurrences (n=40) in each of the eight play contexts and play break per dyad per laugher (N=9 laughers, n=12 play bouts).

In addition, the play context duration of nonlaughers with and without the vocal laughter of their playmates was evaluated (Figure 5). Play context durations of nonlaughers lasted longer when their playmates vocally laughed than when their playmates did not vocally laugh. Although this difference was not significant, it bordered at the threshold of significance (Wilcoxon matched-pairs signed-ranks: Z=1.784; N=10 nonlaughers; p=0.074).

Play initiation

Vocal laughter was never emitted within the last 125 frames (i.e. 5 seconds) prior to the play bout onset. Nor was it ever produced within the first 125 frames after the play bout onset.

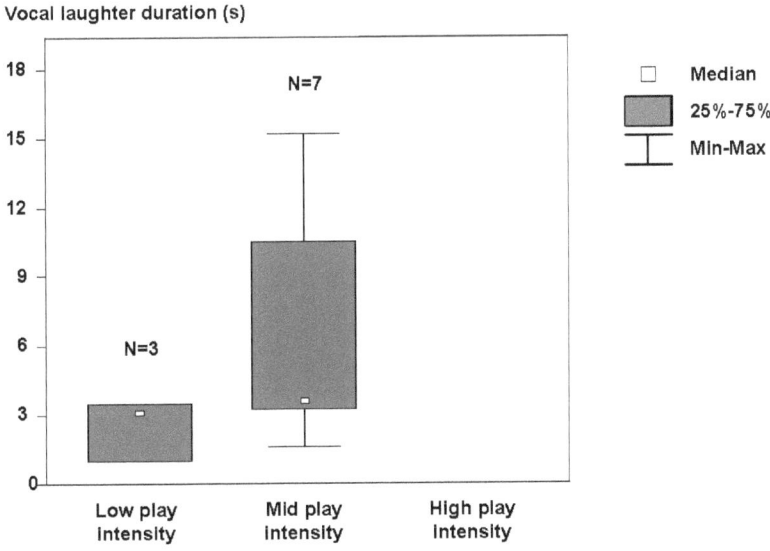

Fig. 3. Vocal laughter duration (n=40) for all three play intensities per dyad per laugher (N=9 laughers, n=12 play bouts). Vocal laughter was present during low (N=3) and mid (N=7) play intensities, but not during high play intensity.

Occurrence of vocal laughter in relation to playmate status: Younger versus older playmates

For Hypothesis 2, Figure 6 depicts vocal laughter frequency of younger and older playmates per dyad per laugher. Neither younger nor older playmates vocally laughed significantly more often (two-tailed Binomial test; N=9 laughers; p=0.100).

Table 6 shows laugher identification of as either younger or older playmates per dyad per laugher.

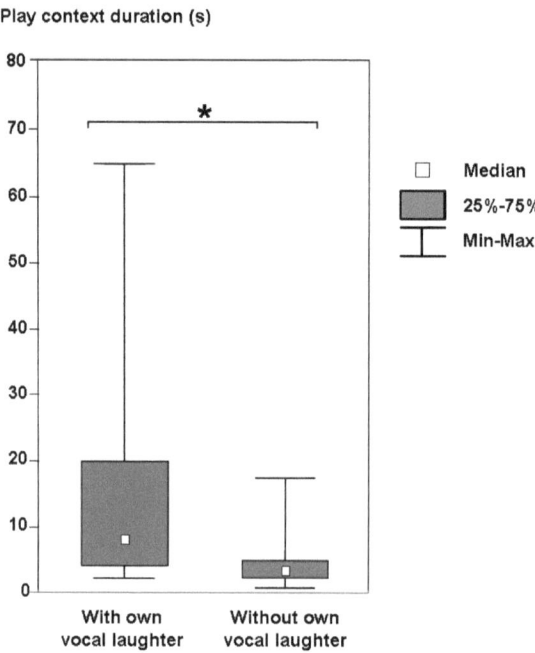

Fig. 4. Play context duration of laughers (N=9) with and without own vocal laughter. These depict a significant difference (Wilcoxon matched-pairs signed-ranks: Z=1.955; p=0.050).

DISCUSSION

In this study, we found that orangutan vocal laughter is neither used more often by younger playmates nor by older playmates. This indicated that orangutan vocal laughter does not signal appeasement to aggressive or fearful playmates, respectively. Furthermore, our data showed tendencies that both playmates continue with the same play actions as before once vocal laughter is emitted by one of the playmates. We also found that orangutan play bouts with vocal laughter lasted longer than those without vocal laughter. In addition, orangutan vocal laughter was evoked during play breaks and, thus, occurred shortly prior to carrying on with play actions. These findings suggested that orangutan vocal laughter represents an expression of arousal/thrill and is used to activate playmates to continue with play. All together, this study on orangutan vocal laughter rejected the Non-aggression and Protection hypotheses, but showed partial support for the Play activation hypothesis.

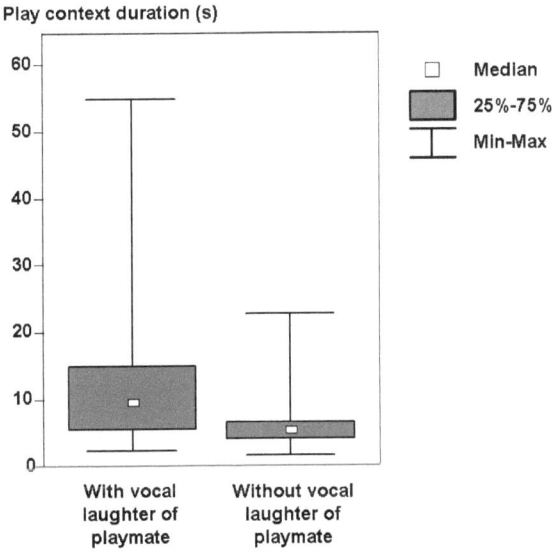

Fig. 5. Play context duration of nonlaughers (N=10) with and without vocal laughter of playmates. Although no significant difference was found, there were tendencies of such difference (Wilcoxon matched-pairs signed-ranks: Z=1.784; p=0.074).

We acknowledged confounding effects that may have been due to the small sample size. However, since orangutans rarely emitted vocal laughter, such could not be avoided despite our large recording collection on orangutan dyadic play.

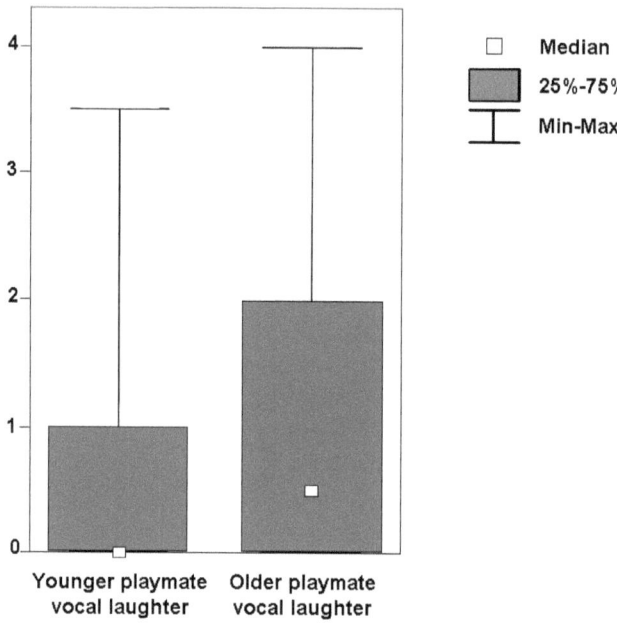

Fig. 6. Vocal laughter frequency of younger and older playmates per dyad per laugher. No significant difference was found (two-tailed Binomial test; N=9 laughers; p=0.100).

Table 6. Laugher identification as either younger or older playmates per dyad per laugher.

Laugher Identification	Laugher as younger playmate	Laugher as older playmate
I4	✸	
I9		✸
I10		✸
J3	✸	
J5		✸
J6	✸	
J7		✸
J8	✸	
S1		✸

Furthermore, different methods used in this study on orangutans and in the study on chimpanzees by Matsusaka (2004) may have caused differences in findings. While Matsusaka (2004) focused on targets and performers of aggressive play, we obtained data only on three dyads during such play. In order to assess all our vocal data, we tested the three vocal laughter hypotheses by comparing either laughers and nonlaughers or younger and older playmates.

Interestingly, vocal laughter is less often produced by orangutans (3.8% of play bouts, this study) than by chimpanzees (39% of play bouts, calculated from Vettin & Todt 2005). Furthermore, orangutans (99% open-mouth faces of 3660 displays including either open-mouth faces or vocal laughter, this study) seem to rely more on facial displays (i.e. open-mouth faces) of the displays including either open-mouth faces or vocal laughter than chimpanzees (83% open-mouth faces of displays including either open-mouth faces or vocal laughter, calculated from Flack et al. 2004). Converged, these inter-specific differences suggest that vocal laughter is less fundamental for orangutan play than for chimpanzee play.

Notably, our data showed that vocal laughter was not used by orangutans to initiate play. Similarly, vocal laughter did not initiate chimpanzee play (Matsusaka 2004).

Since orangutan vocal laughter of this study was never emitted during the highest play intensity, it seems unlikely that it is aroused due to higher play intensity. Particularly, our data on wrestling implied that physical contact is important for a high occurrence of vocal laughter. However, since vocal laughter is also produced during play breaks of no physical contact, orangutan vocal laughter must not be reflexively evoked. Vocal laughter of nontactile games with infant orangutans supported the latter statement (Davila Ross unpubl. data).

Because orangutan laughers continued with their play actions longer than their playmates, our data additionally mirrored that orangutan vocal laughter is a joyous/thrilling expression. For humans, there is strong evidence that hedonic feelings of humor and laughter are linked to activations of the mesolimbic dopaminergic reward system (Mobbs et al. 2003) and that subcortical brain areas, in which the limbic system is located, are shared by all mammals (e.g. reviewed in Panksepp & Burgdorf 2003).

Since social play is essential for self- and social assessment (e.g. Bekoff & Byers 1981) as well as for cognitive development (e.g. Biben 1998), the adaptive value of vocal laughter in orangutans seems to be reflected by its linkage to play bout prolongation. Similar to our results, the ROM display, which categorized to the open-mouth display in this study and which can be accompanied by staccato breathing (i.e. vocal laughter) (e.g. van Hooff 1972), was found to prolong chimpanzee play (Waller & Dunbar 2005). These authors interpreted their results in that relaxed open-mouth displays may reinforce social bonding between playmates.

Conclusively, results of this study revealed that orangutan vocal laughter is not used to appease specific play situations and, therefore, rejected the Non-aggression and Protection hypotheses. Furthermore, our data showed that when orangutan vocal laughter was emitted, play bouts and play actions of both playmates (especially laughers) lasted longer. Thus, these findings suggested that orangutan vocal laughter is used to maintain play and, therefore, rendered partial support for the Play activation hypothesis. Since this was also found in chimpanzees (Matsusaka 2004), there seems to be phylogenetic continuity in the function of vocal laughter to maintain play across great apes.

ACKNOWLEDGMENTS

We are very grateful to S. Nathan, P. Andau, E. Bosi, H. Bernard, and S. Alsisto for their logistic help at Sepilok Orangutan Rehabilitation Centre, to M. Wessels, B. Tia, P. Hristozova, and R. Shockley for their assistance, and to R. Brüning for technical support. The data collection was carried out in Sepilok Orangutan Rehabilitation Centre (SORC). This study was funded by University of Veterinary Medicine Hannover, Center for Systems Neuroscience, Forschungszentrum Jülich GmbH, and Freundeskreis der Tierärztlichen Hochschule Hannover e.V. and was approved by Sabah Wildlife Department and Economic Planning Unit, Malaysia.

REFERENCES

Bekoff, M. & Byers, J.A. 1981 A critical reanalysis of the ontogeny and phylogeny of mammalian social and locomotor play: an ethological hornet's nest. In Behavioral development (eds. K. Immelmann, G. Barlow, M. Main, & L. Petrinovich), pp. 296-337. Cambridge: Cambridge University Press.

Bekoff, M. 1999 Social cognition: exchanging and sharing information on the run. Erkenntnis 51, 113–128.

Berntson, G.G., Boysen, S.T., Bauer, H.R., & Torello M.S. 1989 Conspecific screams and laughter: Cardiac and behavioral reactions of infant chimpanzees. Dev. Psychobiol. 22 (8), 771-787.

Biben, M. 1998 Squirrel monkey play fighting: making the case for a cognitive training function for play. In Animal play: Evolutionary, comparative, and ecological perspectives (eds. M. Bekoff & J.A. Byers), pp. 161-182. Cambridge: Cambridge University Press.

Blurton Jones, N.G. 1967 An ethological study of some aspects of social behaviour of children in nursery school. In Primate ethology (ed. D. Morris). pp 347–368. London: Weidenfeld and Nicolson.

Caron, J.E. 2002 From ethology to aesthetics: Evolution as a theoretical paradigm for research on laughter, humor, and other comic phenomena. Humor 15 (3), 245-281.

Dimberg, U. & Thunberg, M. 1998 Rapid facial reactions to emotional facial expressions. Scand. J. of Psychol. 39, 39-45.

Fagan, R.M. 1981 Animal play behavior. New York: Oxford University Press.

Flack, J.C., Jeannotte, L.A., & de Waal, F.B.M. 2004 Play signaling and the perception of social rules by juvenile chimpanzees (*Pan troglodytes*). J. Comp. Psychol. 118, 149-159.

Fleiss, J.L., Levin, B., & Paik, M.C. 2003 Statistical methods for rates and proportions, 3rd edn. New York: John Wiley & Sons.

Fossey, D. 1983 Gorillas in the mist. Boston: Houghton Mifflin.

Goodall, J. 1986 The chimpanzees of Gombe: Patterns of behavior. Cambridge: Harvard University Press.

Grammer, K. & Eibl-Eibesfeldt, I. 1990 The ritualisation of laughter. In: Natürlichkeit der Sprache und der Kultur (ed. W.A. Koch) pp 192-214. Bochum: Universitätsverlag, Dr. Norbert Brockmeyer.

Harris, C. 1999 The mystery of ticklish laughter. Am. Sci. 87(4), 344-350.

Matsusaka, T. 2004 When does play panting occur during social play in wild chimpanzees? Primates 45, 221-229.

Panksepp, J. & Burgdorf, J. 2003 "Laughing" rats and the evolutionary antecedents of human joy? Physiol.Behav. 79, 533-547.

Preuschoft, S. 1995 'Laughter' and 'smiling' in macaques - an evolutionary perspective. Utrecht: Rijksuniversiteit, 254 p.

Provine, R.R. 1992 Contagious laughter: laughter is a sufficient stimulus for laughs and smiles. Bull. Psychonom. Soc. 30 (1), 1-4.

Provine, R.R. 2000 Laughter: A scientific investigation, New York: Penguin Books.

Rothbart, M.K. 1973 Laughter in young children. Psych. Bull. 80, 247-256.

Rothgänger, H., Hauser, G., Cappelini, A.C., & Guidotti, A. 1998 Analysis of laughter and speech sounds in Italian and German students. Naturwissenschaften 85, 394-402.

Ruvolo, M., Pan, D., Zehr, S., Goldberg, T., Disotell, T.R., & von Dornum, M. 1994 Gene trees and hominoid phylogeny. Proc. Natl. Acad. Sci. USA. 91, 8900-8904.

Sroufe, L.A. & Wunsch, J.P. 1972 The development of laughter in the first year of life. Child Devel. 43,1326-1344.

van Hooff, J.A.R.A.M. & Preuschoft, S. 2003 Laughter and smiling: the intertwining of nature and culture. In Animal social complexity: Intelligence, culture, and individualized societies (eds F.B.M. de Waal & P.L. Tyack), pp 261-287. Cambridge: Harvard University Press.

van Hooff, J.A.R.A.M. 1972 A comparative approach to the phylogeny of laughter and smiling. Non-verbal communication (ed. R. A. Hinde), pp. 209-241. Cambridge: Cambridge University Press.

Vettin, J. & Todt, D. 2005 Human laughter, social play, and play vocalizations of non-human primates: an evolutionary approach. Behaviour 142, 217-240.

Waller, B.M. & Dunbar, R.I.M. 2005 Differential behavioural effects of silent bared teeth display and relaxed open mouth display in chimpanzees (*Pan troglodytes*). Ethology 111, 129-142

Watts, D.P. & Pusey, A.E. 1993 Behavior of juvenile and adolescent great apes. In Juvenile Primates: Life History, Development, and Behavior (eds. M.E. Pereira & L.A. Fairbanks), pp. 148-172. New York: Oxford University Press.

Weisfeld, G.E. 1993 The adaptive value of humor and laughter. Ethol. Sociobiol. 14, 141-169.

CHAPTER 2

RAPID FACIAL MIMICRY IN ORANGUTAN PLAY

INTRODUCTION

Emotional contagion, a subphenomenon of empathy, is a process where individuals express and experience emotions of others. Since it most likely increases individual fitness, it is expected to be phylogenetically continuous (reviewed in Preston & de Waal 2002).

Emotional contagion is closely linked with behavioral congruency (e.g. Hatfield et al. 1994). Since human facial expressions can convey emotions (e.g. Ekman 2003), facial congruency (i.e. mimicry) may provide interesting insights to emotional contagion. Facial congruency was found for various displays of adults, e.g. smiling/laughter (e.g. Lundqvist 1995) and yawning (e.g. Platek et al. 2003), and infants (e.g. Meltzoff & Moore 1997). In humans, rapid facial mimicry (i.e. RFM = facial congruency within 1 second after being exposed to another face) was demonstrated for happy and angry faces (Dimberg & Thunberg 1998). It was argued that RFM involves mainly automatic and reflex-like processes (e.g. Hatfield et al. 1994; Hess & Blairy 2001) inaccessible to conscious awareness (e.g. Dimberg et al. 2000). Alternatively, quick empathic responses may result from neural preparations due to sensory inputs of outer cues (reviewed in Preston & de Waal 2002) and, thereby, include more complex processing mechanisms.

Facial congruency in animals was found for yawning (macaque: Paukner & Anderson 2006; chimpanzee: Anderson et al. 2004) and neonatal imitation (macaque: Ferrari et al. 2006; chimpanzee: e.g. Bard 2006). Findings that specific monkey mirror neurons discharge during the execution and observation of respective facial actions (Ferrari et al. 2003) suggest that facial congruency is also present for various other displays in animals. None of these studies referred to rapidly evoked facial responses.

In this study, we assessed orangutan RFM during social play. Since the human facial expression of laughter, for which nonhuman primate "laugh variants" (i.e. open-mouth faces) were proposed (van Hooff & Preuschoft 2003), can rapidly be mimicked (Dimberg & Thunberg 1998; Dimberg pers. com.), we predicted that RFM is also present for orangutan open-mouth faces (see Table 1 for definition; also see General Introduction, Table 1 for morphological characteristics).

We investigated the occurrence of open-mouth faces that were emitted by both playmates within one second (i.e. bidirectional open-mouth faces or BOMF) for play context, play intensity, and the presence of physical contact in play, respectively. Moreover, because these play components may embody nonfacial factors that could have accounted for RFM-like outcomes, we evaluated the presence of RFM by applying standardizing methods to limit such possible confounding effects. Since the presence of facial congruency may be affected by age (e.g. Myowa-Yamakoshi et al. 2004), we separately assessed RFM for infants and for juveniles and subadults.

METHODS

Data collection, definitions, and videometric analysis

To assess RFM in orangutan social play, a total of 432 dyadic play bouts of 31 orangutans (2-12 years old) were video-recorded ad libitum at Sepilok Orangutan Rehabilitation Centre, Malaysia, Apenheul Primate Park, The Netherlands, and Tierpark Carl Hagenbeck and Zoo Leipzig, Germany. Ontogenetic stages were defined after Watts and Pusey (1993). Data were collected at most playful periods during the day (for 5-8 hours).

Table 1. Definitions of facial displays during orangutan social play.

Facial display	Definition	Example
Open-mouth face	These manifestations represent "laugh variants" of van Hooff and Preuschoft's (2003) study), which included an open-mouth expression of baring no teeth, the relaxed open-mouth (ROM) display, and the relaxed open-mouth bared-teeth (i.e. open-mouth bared-teeth or OMBT) display (also see General Introduction, Table 1 for morphological characteristics). For these displays, lips may be slightly protruding.	
Relaxed face	Neutral face with mouth closed and face muscles relaxed (e.g. van Hooff 1967).	
Nonrelaxed face	Face other than relaxed face (e.g. protruding lips).	

Play involves, according to Fagen (1981), variable, repeated, and/or recombined functional behaviors outside their main contexts. Duration and frequency values were videometrically analyzed with a 3-4 frame resolution using Interact 7.25 (Mangold, Arnstorf, Germany). Dyadic play bout durations began with the first frame when one playmate responded to a play invitation of a second playmate and ended when at least one playmate was not participating for ≥500 frames (i.e. ≥20 seconds) or at the first frame where a third individual interfered. Play breaks were nonplay phases of <500 frames (i.e. <20 seconds) within a play bout.

In addition, facial displays, play contexts, play intensities, and the presence of physical contact during play were videometrically coded for each playmate, respectively. Facial displays were scored either as open-mouth faces, relaxed faces, nonrelaxed faces, transitional faces, and bite faces (see Table 1 for definitions of the three former faces). Transitional faces were intermediaries of open-mouth faces or bite faces and others facial displays. Bite faces were facial manifestations while snapping, chewing, or holding with the jaw the other playmate. Biting is known to take up an important part in nonhuman primate play. Play contexts were defined after Flack et al. (2004) and Vettin and Todt (2005) and were scored either as play with physical contact which included slow grappling, tickling, fast grappling, gnawing, wrestling, hitting, and jumping or as play of no physical contact (see Chapter 1, Table 3 for definitions). In accordance to Flack et al. (2004), the eight play contexts of physical contact in play were grouped into low (slow grappling/tickling), mid (fast grappling/gnawing/wrestling), and high (hitting/jumping) play intensity (see Chapter 1, Table 3). Furthermore, all play contexts of physical contact were grouped and compared to play of no physical contact.

Videos were analyzed by one main observer. Inter-observer reliability was tested by the main and a second observer with one-frame accuracy. Cohen's Kappa results were excellent (Fleiss et al. 2003) with mean agreements of 0.83 for the five facial displays (22 play bouts) and 0.89 for the eight play contexts (21 play bouts), respectively.

Means were used instead of medians if the data values were >5.

BIDIRECTIONAL OPEN-MOUTH FACES

We assessed BOMFs, which occurred when an open-mouth face of one orangutan was followed by an open-mouth face of its playmate within ≤25 frames (≤1 second). Of the 31 orangutans in this study, 25 responded congruently with open-mouth faces of their playmates within this time frame.

In order to assess the occurrence of BOMFs in play contexts, the total numbers of BOMFs (n=152 BOMF events) were scored for each of the eight respective play contexts per individual (N=25). To obtain the percentage of the respective play contexts with BOMFs per individual, these values were divided by their total frequencies per individual and multiplied by 100. Then, mean/median frequency percentages of all individuals were calculated for the respective play contexts. These values were compared across all play contexts, in which BOMF events occurred, using the Chi-square test. The same procedure as above was carried out for the occurrence of BOMFs in play intensities and in the presence of physical contact in play, respectively.

To assess play bout durations with and without BOMFs for each dyad with playmates of the same age group (N=29 dyads), median durations of all play bouts with BOMFs and of all play bouts without BOMFs were calculated per dyad. On the dyad level, play bout durations with BOMFs were compared to play bout durations without BOMFs using the Wilcoxon test.

RFM

Since BOMFs may occur due to factors unrelated to facial mimicry, e.g. physical contact in play, we applied a detailed RFM analysis that excluded confounding variables based on such possible non-facial causes. To test if RFM is present for open-mouth faces in orangutan dyadic play, the facial display of one individual (i.e. subject) was measured as a response to the facial display of another individual (i.e. object). For each subject, the following two scenes were selected: In Object Display, an object produced an open-mouth face; in Object Neutral, the same object produced a neutral face (i.e. nonrelaxed or relaxed faces).

Scenes (i.e. Object Display and Object Neutral) were scored using frame-by-frame analysis for these two facial displays of each of the two playmates, respectively. Scenes were selected according to the following criteria: Both playmates faced each other and the observer needed to identify ≥21 of the coded 25 frames (i.e. 1 second). Furthermore, playmates showed neutral faces at stimulus onsets. Scenes with transitional faces were excluded to avoid possible errors due to uncertainty in coding. Scenes of bite faces, gnawing, and tickling were excluded to reduce possible tickling-like effects, respectively.

Once the first selected video clip was obtained for Object Display, the first video clip we found from a different bout with the same play context was selected for Object Neutral. Thus, scenes could be from any time window within its play bout. Scenes started with the first frame of object facial display and lasted 25 frames.

Since scenes could not be found for six of the recorded orangutans, the sample size for testing RFM was limited to 25 subjects: 10 infants (<4 years old), 11 juveniles (4-9 years old), and 4 subadults (>9 years old).

To test for RFM in infants and juveniles+subadults, the number of congruent reactions and the number of noncongruent reactions of subjects to Object Display and Object Neutral were compared using the Binomial test (see Siegel 1956, pp. 66-67). A congruent reaction occurred when the subject showed an open-mouth face to Object Display (Figure 1) and a neutral face to Object Neutral. A noncongruent reaction occurred when the subject showed a neutral face to Object Display and an open-mouth face in Object Neutral.

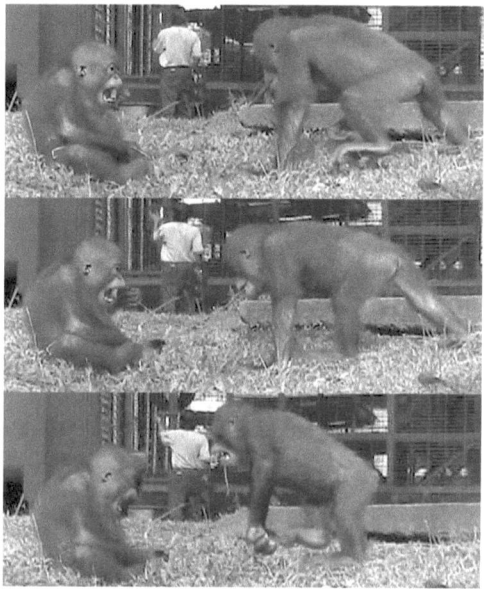

Fig. 1. Open-mouth face of subject (right) to Object Display (left).

By comparing congruent and noncongruent reactions, chance level of open-mouth faces for the studied group was accounted for. If open-mouth faces were produced frequently in Object Neutral, then they were likely to occur with a similar rate in Object Display and would, thus, be statistically ignored.

To measure RFM probability, the total number of subject open-mouth faces in Object Display was subtracted by the total number of subject open-mouth faces in Object Neutral. This value was divided by the total number of subjects and multiplied by 100. RFM probability refers to an absolute increase in probability for subjects displaying open-mouth faces when seeing object open-mouth faces. Probability was calculated after Fleiss et al. (2003).

RESULTS

The occurrence of BOMF events was significantly different across play contexts (Chi-square test: $\chi^2=40.33$; N=6 play contexts; p=0.000), across play intensities (Chi-square test: $\chi^2=47.21$; N=3 play intensities; p=0.000), and between physical contact and no physical contact in play (Chi-square test: $\chi^2=46.80$; N=2 play categories; p=0.000), respectively (Table 2). BOMF occurrences were highest in slow grappling, fast grappling, and wrestling and in mid play intensity and physical contact in play. BOMFs were absent during tickling and jumping.

Table 2. Presence of BOMF events per individual (N=25 subjects, n=152 BOMF events) for play contexts, play intensities, and presence of physical contact in play, respectively. Significant differences were found across play contexts (Chi-square test: $\chi^2=40.33$; N=6 play contexts; p=0.000), across play intensities (Chi-square test: $\chi^2=47.21$; N=3 play intensities; p=0.000), and across physical contact and no physical contact in play (Chi-square test: $\chi^2=46.80$; N=2 play categories; p=0.000).

Play context		Play intensity		Presence of physical contact in play	
Slow grappling (N=7 subjects)	46.73 (n=9)	Low play intensity (N=7 subjects)	46.73 (n=9)	Phys. contact (N=25 subjects)	82.92 (n=148)
Fast grappling (N=22 subjects)	17.84 (n=93)	Mid play intensity (N=22 subjects)	77.79 (n=136)	No phys. contact (N=4 subjects)	15.17 (n=4)
Gnawing (N=6 subjects)	13.87 (n=7)	High play intensity (N=3 subjects)	11.49 (n=3)		
Wrestling (N=13 subjects)	28.91 (n=36)				
Hitting (N=3 subjects)	11.49 (n=3)				
Play of no physical contact (N=4 subjects)	15.17 (n=4)				

Play bout durations with BOMFs were significantly longer than play bout durations without BOMFs (Wilcoxon matched-pairs signed-ranks: Z=2.476; N=29 dyads; p=0.013).

Of the 10 infants, four showed congruent reactions and one showed noncongruent reactions (Figure 2). The number of subjects with congruent reactions and those with noncongruent reactions did not significantly differ (Binomial: N=10, p=0.188). Of the remaining infants, three always produced open-mouth faces and two never produced open-mouth faces. These latter infants were omitted in accordance to the statistical procedure (see methods). The probability of RFM in infant orangutans was 30%.

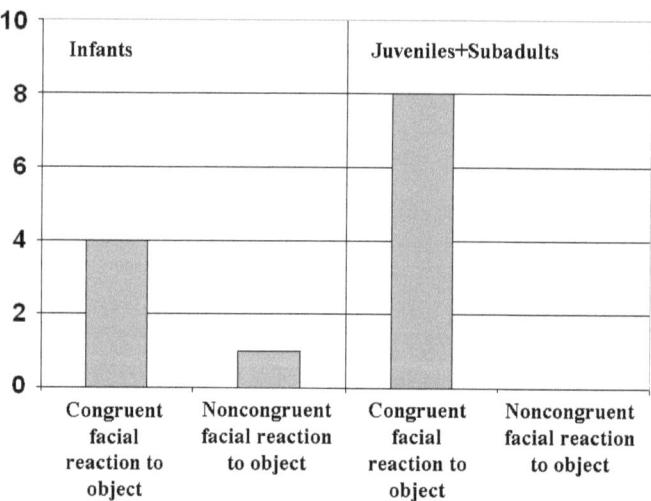

Fig. 2. Number of subjects showing congruent and noncongruent facial reactions to object facial displays. For infant subjects, no significant difference was found (Binomial: N=10 subjects, p=0.188). For juvenile+subadult subjects, a significant difference was found (Binomial: N=15 subjects, p=0.004).

Of the 15 juveniles+subadults, eight showed congruent reactions while no one showed nonconguent reactions (Figure 2). Significantly more juveniles+subadults showed congruent reactions than noncongruent reactions (Binomial: N=15, p=0.004). Concerning the remaining juveniles+subadults, which were statistically omitted by the test (see methods), five consistently produced open-mouth faces and two never emitted these. The probability of RFM in juvenile+subadult orangutans was 53%.

Play vocalizations and hitting were absent throughout all scenes.

DISCUSSION

Our results on RFM for orangutan open-mouth faces demonstrated that infant orangutans did not exhibit congruent reactions significantly more often than noncongruent reactions to their playmates' faces. Contrarily, juvenile+subadult orangutans responded significantly more often congruently than noncongruently to the facial displays of their playmates. Altogether, this study revealed that juveniles and subadults, but not infants, rapidly mimic open-mouth faces of conspecifics in orangutan dyadic play. It provided first evidence on RFM in animals.

We took caution that nonfacial factors, e.g. physical contact in play, may have triggered RFM-like outcomes. Our data on the occurrence of BOMFs indeed indicated that play contexts, play intensities, and presence of physical contact in play may increase the likelihood of RFM-like outcomes. In order to limit these confounding effects, scenes of the same behavioral categories with respect to these factors were selected for each subject in the analytical set-up. Furthermore, the same play constellations were used for each subject. And play vocalizations, play biting, tickling, gnawing, jumping, and hitting were entirely absent throughout all scenes. Due to this equivalence across compared scenes, we found it unlikely that our findings on RFM were the directly affected by nonfacial cues.

Our data revealed that play bouts with BOMFs lasted longer than those without BOMFs. Similarly, Waller and Dunbar (2005) found that chimpanzee play bouts lasted longer if both playmates emitted relaxed open-mouth (i.e. ROM) displays than if just one playmate emitted such a facial display during play. The ROM display is a component of the open-mouth face in this study. Like Waller and Dunbar (2005), we presumed that such bidirectional behaviors indicated that these facial displays represent both playmates' motivation to play. Such motivation could lead to a prolongation in play.

Since great ape ROM displays are perceived as positive signals by conspecifics (e.g. Parr 2001) and serve social cohesion (Waller & Dunbar 2005), we suggest that by displaying open-mouth faces during play, orangutans evoke the same positive emotions in their playmates. This way, RFM represents a component of emotional contagion. Like other empathic mechanisms (Preston & de Waal 2002), facial mimicry may facilitate social bonding, which may, thus, reinforce cooperative systems.

Although it could be that orangutans also use nonrapid facial mimicry, which would most likely involve voluntary congruency, we focused in this study on RFM. RFM refers mainly to programmed responses (e.g. Dimberg & Thunberg 1998). However, our results revealed that there are other factors that may additionally affect RFM. Strong support comes from our findings on RFM across age groups. Since infants (2-4 years of age) showed no RFM, unlike juveniles and subadults, our results implied that there is an impact of experience on RFM.

Furthermore, our RFM probability results indicated that 47% of the times, open-mouth faces did not trigger facial congruency in juvenile and subadult orangutans.

We proposed the following two explanations for this. Firstly, certain open-mouth faces, e.g. OMBT displays, may be more likely to cause RFM than others. Secondly, open-mouth faces, which occur in the socio-positive contexts of play, might be superimposed by socio-emotional factors, e.g. by playing with a favorite playmate. In humans, socio-emotional factors influence laughter congruency (e.g. Freedman & Perlick 1979) and various other empathic processes (e.g. Decety & Jackson 2006).

Conclusively, this study showed that rapid open-mouth face mimicry is present in juvenile and subadult orangutans. Since we found no such evidence on infant orangutans, our data suggested that RFM can be affected by experience. Furthermore, the presence of RFM may be influenced by specific play contexts, play intensities, and the presence of physical contact. Altogether, our results implied that ape RFM can be processed via diverse integral compounds of affective communication, which show strong parallels to fundamental building blocks of emotional contagion and empathy in man.

ACKNOWLEDGMENTS

Thanks go to S. Nathan, P. Andau, E. Bosi, H. Bernard for logistic help, to U. Radespiel for advice, and to M. Wessels, B. Tia, R. Shockley, C. Schopf, and R. Brüning for assistance. Data collection was supported by MPI for Evolutionary Anthropology Leipzig, Sabah Wildlife Department, Sepilok Orangutan Rehabilitation Centre (SORC), Apenheul Primate Park, Tierpark Carl Hagenbeck, and Zoo Leipzig. Research was funded by University of Veterinary Medicine Hannover, Center for Systems Neuroscience Hannover, Forschungszentrum Jülich GmbH, and Freundeskreis der Tierärztlichen Hochschule Hannover e.V.

REFERENCES

Anderson, J.R., Myowa-Yamakoshi, M., & Matsuzawa, T. 2004 Contagious yawning in chimpanzees. Proc. R. Soc. B 271, 468-470.

Bard, K. 2006 Neonatal imitation in chimpanzees (*Pan troglodytes*) tested with two paradigms. Anim. Cogn.

Decety, J. & Jackson, P.L. 2006 A social-neuroscience perspective on empathy. Curr. Direct. Psychol. Sci. 15 (2), 54–58.

Dimberg, U., Thunberg, M. & Elmehed, K. 2000 Unconscious facial reactions to emotional facial expressions. Psychol. Sci. 11, 86-89.

Dimberg, U. & Thunberg, M. 1998 Rapid facial reactions to emotional facial expressions. Scand. J. of Psychol. 39, 39-45.

Ekman, P. 2003 Emotions Revealed: recognizing faces and feelings to improve communication and emotional life. New York: Times Books

Fagan, R.M. 1981 Animal play behavior. New York: Oxford University Press.

Ferrari, P.F., Gallese, V., Rizzolatti, G., & Fogassi, L. 2003 Mirror neurons responding to the observation of ingestive and communicative mouth actions in the monkey ventral premotor cortex. Eur. J. Neurosci. 17 (8), 1703–1714.

Ferrari, P.F., Visalberghi, E., Paukner, A., Fogassi, L., Ruggiero, A., Suomi, S.J. 2006 Neonatal imitation in rhesus macaques. PLoS Biol. 4(9), e302.

Flack, J.C., Jeannotte, L.A., & de Waal, F.B.M. 2004 Play signaling and the perception of social rules by juvenile chimpanzees (*Pan troglodytes*). J. Comp. Psychol. 118, 149-159.

Fleiss, J.L., Levin, B., & Paik, M.C. 2003 Statistical methods for rates and proportions, 3rd edn. New York: John Wiley & Sons.

Freedman, J.L. & Perlick, D. 1979 Crowding, contagion, and laughter. J. Exp. Soc. Psychol 15, 295-303.

Hatfield, E., Cacioppo, J.T. & Rapson, R.L. 1994 Emotional contagion, Cambridge: Cambridge University Press.

Hess, U. & Blairy, S. 2001 Facial mimicry and emotional contagion to dynamic emotional facial expressions and their influence on decoding accuracy. Int. J. Psychophysiol. 40, 129-141.

Lundqvist, L.-O. 1995 Facial EMG reactions to facial expressions: A case of facial emotional contagion? Scand. J. of Psychol. 36, 130-141.

Meltzoff, A.N. & Moore, M.K. 1997 Explaining facial imitation: A theoretical model. Early Dev. Parenting 6, 179-192.

Myowa-Yamakoshi, M., Tomonaga, M., Tanaka, M., & Matsuzawa, T. 2004 Imitation in neonatal chimpanzees (*Pan troglodytes*). Dev. Sci. 7(4), 437-442

Parr, L.A. 2001 Cognitive and physiological markers of emotional awareness in chimpanzees (*Pan troglodytes*). Anim. Cogn. 4, 223-229.

Paukner, A. & Anderson, J.R. 2006 Video-induced yawning in stumptail macaques (*Macaca arctoides*). Biol. Lett. 2, 36-38.

Platek, S.M., Critton, S.R., Myers, T.E. & Gallup G.G. 2003 Contagious yawning: The role of self-awareness and mental state attribution. Cogn. Brain Res. 17, 223-227.

Preston, S.D. & de Waal, F.B.M. 2002 Empathy: Its ultimate and proximate bases. Behav. Brain Sci. 25, 1-72.

Siegel, S. 1956 Nonparametric statistics for the behavioral sciences, 1st edn. New York: McGraw-Hill Book Company.

van Hooff, J.A.R.A.M. & Preuschoft, S. 2003 Laughter and smiling: The intertwining of nature and culture. In Animal Social Complexity: Intelligence, culture, and individualized societies (eds F.B.M. de Waal & P.L. Tyack), pp 261-287. Cambridge: Harvard University Press.

van Hooff, J.A.R.A.M. 1967 The facial displays of the Catarrhine monkeys and apes. In Primate Ethology (ed. D. Morris), pp. 7-68. London: Weidenfeld and Nicholson.

Vettin, J. & Todt, D. 2005 Human laughter, social play, and play vocalizations of non-human primates: an evolutionary approach. Behaviour 142, 217-240.

Waller, B.M. & Dunbar, R.I.M. 2005 Differential behavioural effects of silent bared teeth display and relaxed open mouth display in chimpanzees (*Pan troglodytes*). Ethology 111, 129-142.

Watts, D.P. & Pusey, A.E. 1993 Behavior of juvenile and adolescent great apes. In Juvenile Primates: Life History, Development, and Behavior (eds. M.E. Pereira & L.A. Fairbanks), pp. 148-172. New York: Oxford University Press.

CHAPTER 3

TOWARDS THE EVOLUTIONARY ORIGIN OF VOCAL LAUGHTER — A COMPARATIVE ACOUSTIC AND PHYLOGENETIC ANALYSIS ON TICKLING VOCALIZATIONS OF GREAT APES AND HUMANS

INTRODUCTION

Vocal laughter is an important component of nonverbal emotional and semantic communication in humans. However, despite the many studies on various aspects of human vocal laughter (e.g. arousal: e.g. Sroufe & Wunsch 1972; contagion: e.g. Freedman & Perlick 1978; conversation: Vettin & Todt 2004; humor: e.g. Gervais & Wilson 2005; tickling: e.g. Harris 1999), its biological roots are still poorly understood. Studies on humans revealed that vocal laughter is a cross-cultural phenomenon (e.g. Ekman 1973) and can be emitted by newborns (e.g. Scheiner et al. 2002) and deaf-blind children (e.g. Eibl-Eibesfeldt 1985). These findings indicated that vocal laughter may have a prehuman basis.

Of the vocal repertoire in nonhuman primates, vocalizations emitted during play most evidently show contextual similarities with human vocal laughter. Play signals, such as play vocalizations, can serve different functions in mammalian play, e.g. to maintain social play (e.g. Bekoff 1995) or invite to play (e.g. Fagen 1981). Since social play embodies a foundation for self- and social assessment (e.g. Bekoff & Byers 1981) and cognitive development (e.g. Biben 1998) and, thus, supports cooperative systems (e.g. Fagen 1981), play vocalizations are fundamental tools for social species and, as such, could have evolved more than once. Indeed, they are ubiquitous in mammalian play (e.g. galagos: Zimmermann 1989, 1991; loris: e.g. Zimmermann 1991; mouse lemurs: Zimmermann 1995; tamarins: e.g. Cleveland & Snowdon 1982; howler monkeys: e.g. Baldwin & Baldwin 1976; colobus: e.g. Struhsaker 1975; dogs: Robbins & McCreery 2003; rats: Panksepp & Burgdorf 2003). Concerning hominoids, acoustically distinct types of play vocalizations were observed in orangutans (e.g. Rijksen 1978) and humans (e.g. Scheiner et al. 2002). Thus, caution needs to be taken when generalizing animal play vocalizations as phylogenetic precursors of human vocal laughter (e.g. "laughing" rats: Panksepp & Burgdorf 2003).

Similar to human vocal laughter (e.g. Harris 1999), tickling can evoke low-frequency (LF) vocalizations in all apes (white-handed gibbons: Zimmermann pers. obs.; siamangs: Geissmann pers. com.; orangutans: Chevalier-Skolnikoff 1982; gorillas: Schenkel 1964; chimpanzees: e.g. van Hooff & Preuschoft 2003; bonobos: Förderreuther & Zimmermann 2003). Tickling is a component of social play in great apes (e.g. Fossey 1983; Goodall 1986) where relaxed open-mouth displays (e.g. van Hooff, 1972) and "laughing" expressions (i.e. open-mouth bared-teeth displays) frequently occur (e.g. de Waal 1988). These facial expressions were proposed to represent "laugh variants" (Preuschoft 1995; van Hooff & Preuschoft 2003). Commonality in the sound-releasing context of tickling between great ape LF tickling vocalizations and human vocal laughter suggests homology, i.e. an "inferred common ancestry" (Patterson 1988). Compatible with this, chimpanzee vocalizations of tickling or play and human vocal laughter are similar in intra- and inter-individual acoustic variability (Vettin & Todt 2005). Furthermore, like human vocal laughter, vocalizations of chimpanzees (e.g. van Hooff 1972) and bonobos (e.g. de Waal 1988) during tickling or play show a staccato rhythm. Despite of these commonalities, the phylogenetic relationship between great ape LF tickling vocalizations and human vocal laughter during tickling, which may provide important insights to the evolution of vocal laughter in humans, was never explored.

In this study, we tested for phylogenetic continuity in LF tickling vocalizations of orangutan, gorilla, chimpanzee, bonobo, and human infants and young juveniles. Because they all share the same sound-releasing context and a comparable sound production mechanism (e.g. Fitch 2000), we postulated that these vocalizations of great apes and humans are homologous. Homology would be supported if a phylogenetic tree based on tickling-elicited LF vocalizations was found to be congruent with the widely accepted topology of hominoids based on genetics (e.g. McBrearty & Jablongski 2005; Ruvolo et al. 1994; Wildman et al. 2002) (see General Introduction, Figure 5). We tested our hypothesis by applying an acoustic and phylogenetic analysis of these vocalizations across the five hominoid taxa.

For this study, we chose infants and young juveniles to limit confounding effects by vocal learning (chimpanzees: e.g. Marshall et al. 1999; bonobos: Taglialatela et al. 2003; humans: e.g. Locke et al. 1995) and developmental changes of the larynx position throughout ontogeny (chimpanzees: e.g. Nishimura et al. 2003; humans: e.g. Lieberman et al. 2001).

METHODS

Data collection

During tickling sessions, LF tickling vocalizations of the following hominoid taxa were recorded: Siamang (N=1 individual), orangutan (N=7), gorilla (N=5), chimpanzee (N=4), bonobo (N=5), and human (N=3). These subjects were mostly tickled at their palms, feet, armpits, and necks, since LF tickling vocalizations were most easily evoked this way. Tickling sessions were conducted by known ticklers and in facilities familiar to subjects.

Subjects were 6-56 months old. Table 1 depicts information on age, gender, rearing, recorder, recording equipment, tickler identification, tickling facility, and digitizing procedure.

Spectrographic examples of LF tickling vocalizations of each taxon are shown in Figure 1.

Acoustic analyses

Sounds of wav. format were converted to ESPS format and downsampled from the original sampling rate to 22050 Hz (see Table 1 for original sampling rates). A high-pass 60Hz-region filter was applied to remove energy that could have resulted in alternating current fluctuations. Start times were reset to 0.0 seconds. Any possible direct-current offsets due to tape-recording artifacts were removed to center the waveform to the zero-voltage line. The full width of the amplitude scale was scaled. We used the 5.3 x-waves software (Entropic Research Lab, Washington, DC).

All recordings with a difference of <2dB between calls and background noise were omitted from further analysis. The total numbers of analyzed calls per subject are presented in Table 1.

All sounds were measured at FFT-based narrowband spectrogram (40-ms Hanning window), spectral slice, waveform, and wideband spectrogram (8-ms Hanning window) with preemphasis of 0.94 (see Table 2).

Table 1. Studied subjects with information on age, gender, rearing, number of analyzed calls, recorder, recording equipment, tickler identification, tickling facility, and digitizing procedure.

Taxon	Ind. ID	Age & gender	Rear.	No.[1] of calls	Recorder & Recording equipment[1]	Tickler identification & facility	Sampling rate, resolution, & digitizing software
Siamang[2]	S1	54 mo; male	Parent-reared	21	MDR; TR: Sony WM-D6C, d-mic: Sennheiser ME 60	Caretaker at Zoo Berlin, Germany	44kHz/16 bit; PRAAT 4.5[4]
Orangutan	O1	6 mo; male	Peer-reared	24	BF; TR: Nagra IV-SJ, d-mic: Sennheiser MKH 816	Caretaker at Wilhelma, Stuttgart, Germany	22kHz/16 bit; Batsound Pro 3.31[3]
	O2	11 mo; female	Peer-reared	10	BF; TR: Nagra IV-SJ, d-mic: Sennheiser MKH 816	Caretaker at Wilhelma, Stuttgart, Germany	22kHz/16 bit; Batsound Pro 3.31[3]
	O3	22 mo; male	Peer-reared	9	BF; TR: Nagra IV-SJ, d-mic: Sennheiser MKH 816	Caretaker at Wilhelma, Stuttgart, Germany	22kHz/16 bit; Batsound Pro 3.31[3]
	O4	24 mo; male	Peer-reared	3	MDR; TR: Sony WM-D6C, d-mic: Sennheiser ME 60	Caretaker at Wilhelma, Stuttgart, Germany	44kHz/16 bit; PRAAT 4.5[4]
	O5	30 mo; male	Peer-reared	11	MDR; TR: Sony WM-D6C, d-mic: Sennheiser ME 60	MDR at SORC[1], Malaysia	44kHz/16 bit; PRAAT 4.5[4]
	O6	36 mo; female	Peer-reared	11	MDR; TR: Sony WM-D6C, d-mic: Sennheiser ME 60	MDR at SORC[1], Malaysia	44kHz/16 bit; PRAAT 4.5[4]
	O7	42 mo; male	Peer-reared	69	MDR; TR: Sony WM-D6C, d-mic: Sennheiser ME 60	MDR at SORC[1], Malaysia	40kHz/16 bit; PRAAT 4.5[4]
Gorilla	G1	6 mo; female	Peer-reared	25	MDR; TR: Sony WM-D6C, d-mic: Sennheiser ME 60	Caretaker at Wilhelma, Stuttgart, Germany	44kHz/16 bit; PRAAT 4.5[4]
	G2	10 mo; female	Peer-reared	35	MDR; TR: Sony WM-D6C, d-mic: Sennheiser ME 60	Caretaker at Wilhelma, Stuttgart, Germany	44kHz/16 bit; PRAAT 4.5[4]
	G3	11 mo; female	Peer-reared	45	BF; TR: Nagra IV-SJ, d-mic: Sennheiser MKH 816	Caretaker at Wilhelma, Stuttgart, Germany	22kHz/16 bit; Batsound Pro 3.31[3]
	G4	30 mo; female	Peer-reared	17	MDR; TR: Sony WM-D6C, d-mic: Sennheiser ME 60	Caretaker at Wilhelma, Stuttgart, Germany	44kHz/16 bit; PRAAT 4.5[4]
	G5	42 mo; female	Parent-reared	24	MDR; TR: Sony WM-D6C, d-mic: Sennheiser ME 60	Caretaker at Zoo Berlin, Germany	44kHz/16 bit; PRAAT 4.5[4]
Chimpanzee	C1	8 mo; male	Parent-reared	30	BF; TR: Nagra IV-SJ, d-mic: Sennheiser MKH 816	Caretaker at Zoo Hannover, Germany	22kHz/16 bit; Batsound Pro 3.31[3]
	C2	10 mo; male	Parent-reared	95	BF; TR: Nagra IV-SJ, d-mic: Sennheiser MKH 816	Caretaker at Zoo Hannover, Germany	22kHz/16 bit; Batsound Pro 3.31[3]
	C3	11 mo; female	Parent-reared	99	BF; TR: Nagra IV-SJ, d-mic: Sennheiser MKH 816	Caretaker at Schwaben Park, Kaiserbach, Germany	22kHz/16 bit; Batsound Pro 3.31[3]
	C4	20 mo; male	Peer-reared	31	BF; TR: Nagra IV-SJ, d-mic: Sennheiser MKH 816	Caretaker at Schwaben Park, Kaiserbach, Germany	22kHz/16 bit; Batsound Pro 3.31[3]
Bonobo	B1	9 mo; male	Peer-reared	149	BF; TR: Nagra IV-SJ, d-mic: Sennheiser MKH 816	Caretaker at Zoo Wuppertal, Germany	44kHz/16 bit; Batsound Pro 3.31[3]
	B2	11 mo; female	Parent-reared	16	MDR; TR: Sony WM-D6C, d-mic: Sennheiser ME 60	Caretaker at Apenheul Primate Park, Apeldoorn, The Netherlands	44kHz/16 bit; PRAAT 4.5[4]
	B3	33 mo; female	Peer-reared	20	BF; TR: Nagra IV-SJ, d-mic: Sennheiser MKH 816	Caretaker at Wilhelma, Stuttgart, Germany	22kHz/16 bit; Batsound Pro 3.31[3]
	B4	45 mo; male	Peer-reared	8	BF; TR: Nagra IV-SJ, d-mic: Sennheiser MKH 816	Caretaker at Zoo Frankfurt, Germany	22kHz/16 bit; Batsound Pro 3.31[3]
	B5	56 mo; female	Peer-reared	11	BF; TR: Nagra IV-SJ, d-mic: Sennheiser MKH 816	Caretaker at Wilhelma, Stuttgart, Germany	22kHz/16 bit; Batsound Pro 3.31[3]
Human	H1	11 mo; male	Parent-reared	13	MDR; TR: Sony WM-D6C, d-mic: Sennheiser ME 60	Mother at private home, Germany	22kHz/16 bit; PRAAT 4.5[4]
	H2	12 mo; male	Parent-reared	29	MDR; TR: Sony WM-D6C, d-mic: Sennheiser ME 60	Mother at private home, Germany	22kHz/16 bit; PRAAT 4.5[4]
	H3	19 mo; female	Parent-reared	6	MDR; TR: Sony WM-D6C, d-mic: Sennheiser ME 60	Mother at private home, Germany	22kHz/16 bit; PRAAT 4.5[4]

[1] Abbreviations: BF=B. Förderreuther; d-=directional; Ind. ID=individual identification; MDR=M. Davila Ross; mic=microphone; No.=number; Rear.=rearing; SORC=Sepilok Orangutan Rehabilitation Centre; SR=sampling rate; TR=tape-recorder.
[2] Outgroup of phylogenetic analysis
[3] Pettersson Elektronik AB, Uppsala, Sweden
[4] Paul Boersma & David Weenink, Amsterdam, The Netherlands

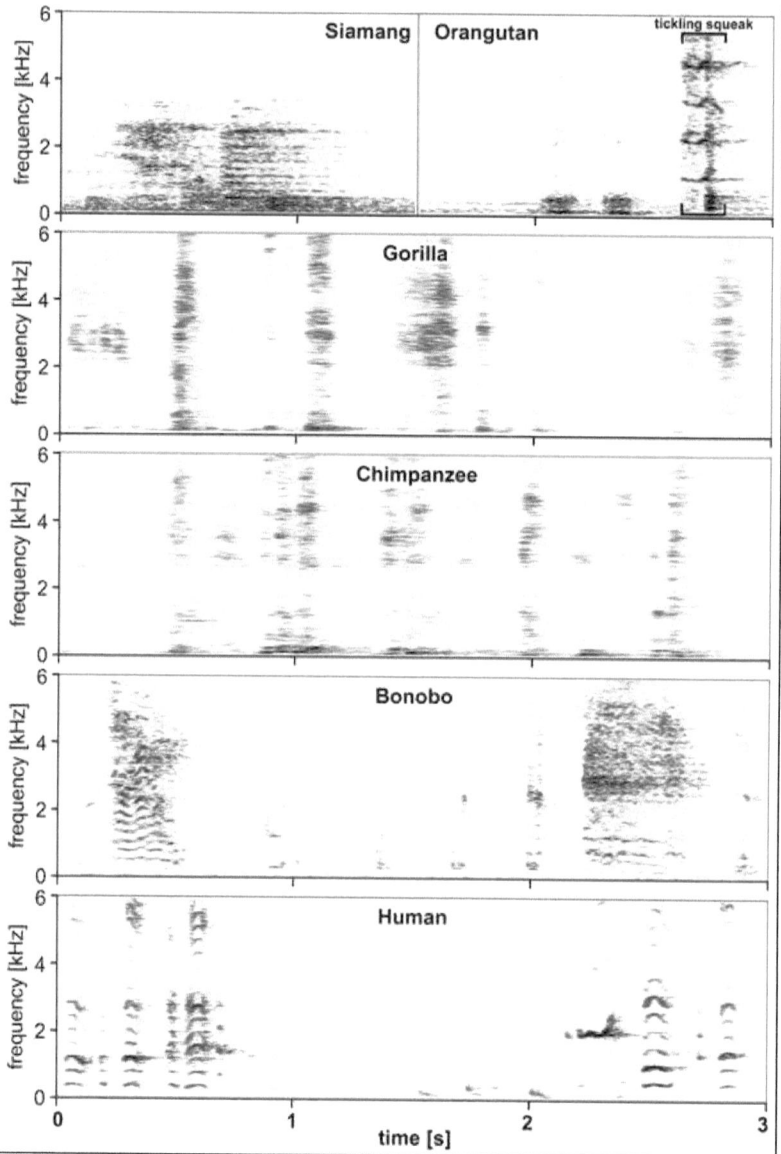

Fig. 1. Spectrograms of siamang, orangutan, gorilla, chimpanzee, and bonobo LF tickling vocalizations, human vocal laughter, and orangutan HF tickling vocalizations, i.e. tickling squeaks.

Table 2. Terms, definitions, and ranges of individuals for each hierarchical level (call segment, call, bout, bout series) and acoustic variable. Altogether, four hierarchical levels and 16 acoustic variables were assessed. Every sound was measured using narrowband spectrograms (n) (40-ms Hanning window), spectral slices (s), waveforms (v), and wideband spectrograms (w) (8-ms Hanning window) with preemphasis of 0.94.

ID[1]	Sound level & variable	Units	Definition and ranges of individuals[2]
	Call segment		**Acoustic element within a call consisting of specific degrees of periodicity (noise, deterministic chaos, tonality).**
1	Segment noise	%	Presence of aperiodic irregular vibrations showing a broadband spectrum of equal energy distribution within a frequency range of >2 kHz over its absence (nsvw); in accordance to e.g. Fitch et al. (2002).
2	Segment deterministic chaos	%	Presence of deterministic chaos (aperiodic vibrations showing broadband spectrum of unequal energy distribution of >2 kHz), of biphonation (sidebands measured after ≥3 amplitude modulations; 2 independently moving oscillators measured at ≤2 kHz and ≥3 kHz frequency ranges) accenting in deterministic chaos, and of residuary regularity (pseudoharmonics showing periodic patterns at three or more frequency levels; subharmonics present as multiples of 1/2) accenting in deterministic chaos over its absence (nsvw); in accordance to e.g. Fitch et al. (2002), Riede et al. (1997, 2004), and Tokuda et al. (2002).
3	Segment tonality	%	Presence of dominant periodic structures over its absence (nsvw); in accordance to e.g. Fischer et al. (2001).
	Call		**Continuous sound element over time without sound gap that shows abrupt energy boost and decline at its start and end points, respectively.**
4	Segments/call		Number of call segments per call (vw).
5	Call duration	s	Duration from start to end of call (vw).
6	Call rhythm	s	Duration from start of one call to start of successive call (vw).
7	Spectral slope		Spectral slope measured at call midway (s).
8	1st spectral moment	Hz	Mean of spectral moment measured at call midway (s); in accordance to Boersma and Weenink (2007).
9	2nd spectral moment	Hz	Standard deviation of spectral moment measured at call midway (s); in accordance to Boersma and Weenink (2007).
10	Call peak frequency	Hz	Frequency with highest peak amplitude measured at call midway (s).
	Bout		**Consecutive calls of the same mode (i.e. either calls of same rhythm, same duration, or same phenotype) or consecutive calls with an interval duration of <8 milliseconds.**
11	Rhythm pattern	%	Presence of bouts with calls of same rhythm over their absence (vw).
12	Phenotype pattern	%	Presence of bouts with calls of same phenotype over their absence (nvw).
13	Contiguity pattern	%	Presence of bouts with calls of interval duration of <8 milliseconds over their absence (vw).
14	Alternating respiration	%	Presence of bouts with calls alternating in exhalation-inhalation patterns over their absence (vw).
	Bout series		**Group of consecutive bouts with an interbout interval of < 1 second.**
15	Calls/series		Number of calls per bout series (vw).
16	Bouts/series		Number of bouts per bout series (vw).

[1] Variable identification number
[2] for phylogenetic analysis

LF tickling vocalizations were measured at four hierarchical sound levels (see Table 2 for definitions): Call segment, call, bout, and bout series (see Figure 2 for scheme). The acoustics of call segments were categorized with regard to different degrees of periodicity: Noise, deterministic chaos, and tonality (see Table 2 for definitions). Spectrographic examples of these are depicted in Figure 3.

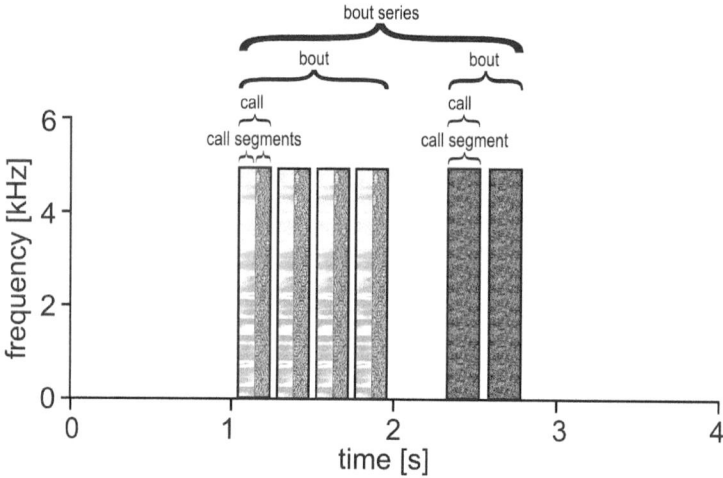

Fig. 2. Scheme of the four hierarchical sound levels: Call segment, call, bout, and bout series.

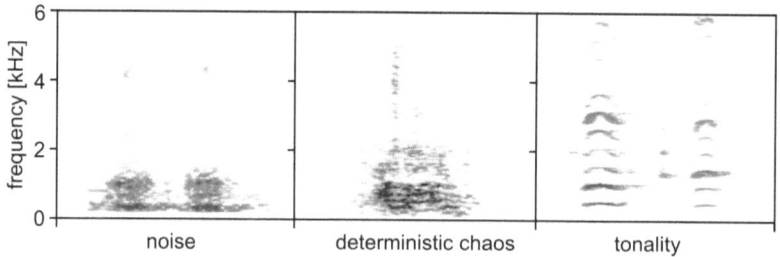

Fig. 3. Examples of noise, deterministic chaos, and tonality in spectrogram.

A total of 16 acoustic variables, that were measured in accordance to the four hierarchical sounds levels, were obtained (see Table 2 for definitions of acoustic variables).

The 1st and 2nd spectral moments (variables 8 and 9, respectively) mark speaker identification in humans (Eriksson et al. 2004; Rodman et al. 2002).

A phenotype represented the energy distribution over time in a narrowband and wideband spectrogram (see Table 2). The term "same" in "same rhythm" for rhythm pattern (variable 11) and "same phenotype" for phenotype pattern (variable 12) referred to commonalities in every call, in every second call, or in every third call of all sequential calls per bout (see Table 2).

Bouts consisted either of alternating exhalation-inhalation calls or consecutive exhalation calls. Therefore, the definition of alternating respiration (variable 14) does not include consecutive inhalation calls (see Table 2).

All recordings were measured by MDR. For identifying calls of exhalation and inhalation (variable 14), only calls with respiration types found in agreement between the main and a second analyzer were included for further analyses. Of all measured calls, 11% were omitted due to either disagreement or uncertainty of labelling the calls.

For each individual, medians or means were first of all calculated for all call segments within each call, then for all calls within each bout, for all bouts within each bout series, and for all bout series. If the number of data values was ≤5, medians were used. If the number of data values were >5, means were calculated. On the taxon level, medians across individuals were used to avoid outlier effects (Tabachnick & Fidell 2006).

For comparisons across the four great apes and humans, Chi-square tests and one-way ANOVA's were applied for nominal (N=10; variables 1-4, & 11-16) and ordinal (N=6; variables 5-10) data sets of every variable, respectively, using STATISTICA 6.1 (StatSoft, Tulsa, OK, USA). For these analyses, α-adjustments were made applying the Hommel-Hochberg correction (Hochberg & Hommel 1998). Post hoc tests were Chi-square tests and Mann-Whitney U test for the respective analyses. For these tests, once again the Hommel-Hochberg correction was applied.

Phylogenetic analyses

Siamang (i.e. outgroup) LF tickling vocalizations were used to root the phylogenetic tree of great ape and human (i.e. ingroup) LF tickling vocalizations (Table 1). Outgroup data were measured with the same methods as ingroup data.

For each variable, subject means were standardized with log (x+1) transformations (Thiele 1993). Medians across subjects were calculated for each variable of each taxon.

Data of all variables or characters were coded in accordance to the gap-weighting method by Thiele (1993). Garcia-Cruz & Sosa (2006) demonstrated that the gap-weighting method performed better than four alternative approaches for coding continuous data in phylogenetic analyses based on the criteria for accuracy discussed by Wiens (1995). The gap-weighting method weighs gaps between coded states (character states) of two taxa differently by giving larger weights to larger differences in their trait averages. For this study, 10 character states were selected after Thiele (1993).

For the phylogenetic reconstruction, the exhaustive search and bootstrap analyses were implemented by PAUP* 4.0b10 (PPC) software (Swofford, Sinauer Associates, Sunderland, MA, USA). Exhaustive search is a method that shows a consensus of the most parsimonious trees (e.g. Maddison & Madisson 2000). Bootstrap analysis was used for assessing the support of clades (e.g. Felsenstein

1985). Such support was represented by bootstrap values for a consensus of tree replications (Kitching et al. 1998). In this study, 1000 replications according to Archangelsky (2004) and Robillard et al. (2006) were generated.

For tree and character diagnostics, treelength, consistency index (CI), and retention index (RI) were calculated in PAUP. The treelength expresses the total number of evolutionary steps of every character in a phylogenetic tree (e.g. Swofford 1990). The smaller the treelength, the better data fit the tree. CI measures the degree of homoplasy or character states evolving more than once in a clade (e.g. Kitching et al. 1998). RI shows the amount of synapomorphies or collectively derived character states in a clade (Farris 1989). For both indices, values close to 1 (range of 0 to 1) show close to no homoplasy.

For characters with CI≥0.900 and RI≥0.900, character state tracings of individual character evolution was conducted using MacClade 4.0 (Maddison & Maddison, Sinauer Associates, Sunderland, MA, USA). Characters of these qualities were considered to show strongest support for the resulting tree.

RESULTS

Acoustic comparison of tickling vocalizations across taxa

Besides LF tickling vocalizations, high-frequency (HF) tickling vocalizations were heard in orangutans and humans during tickling. In orangutans, HF tickling vocalizations, i.e. tickling squeaks, were more frequent than LF tickling vocalizations (see Figure 1, for spectrogram of orangutan tickling squeak).

Taxon medians of all 16 variables are depicted in Table 3.

Table 3. Medians and ranges (in parentheses) of all hominoids (S, O, G, C, B, H)[1], results of Chi-square tests and one-way ANOVA's for taxon-specific comparisons, and indices of character diagnostics of the exhaustive search for the 16 acoustic variables. The characters with CI≥0.900 and RI≥0.900 are marked bold.

ID[2]	S[3]	O	G	C	B	H	Chi-square test (N=5)	one-way ANOVA (N=5)	Exhaustive search
1	71.296	52.083 (0-67.740)	41.817 (33.33-79.167)	47.844 (30.561-66.204)	37.582 (19.444-43.229)	12.761 (0-25.000)	χ^2=619.606; p<0.000		CI=0.900; RI=0.500
2	28.704	22.917 (6.466-50.000)	52.153 (20.833-58.833)	49.857 (31.019-67.629)	50.926 (25.521-58.333)	27.997 (27.111-33.333)	χ^2=656.227; p<0.000		CI=0.562; RI=0.462
3	0	0	0	0	0 (0-0.202)	72.556 (50.000-100.000)	χ^2=290.222; p<0.000		CI=1.000; RI=0/0
4	**1.388**	**1.333 (1.261-2.100)**	**1.556 (1.000-1.815)**	**1.510 (1.100-1.802)**	**1.5 (1.219-2.069)**	**2.333 (1.487-2.486)**	**χ^2=26.419; p<0.000**		**CI=1.000; RI=1.000**
5	**0.137**	**0.139 (0.118-0.310)**	**0.138 (0.123-0.206)**	**0.080 (0.059-0.096)**	**0.095 (0.068-0.191)**	**0.087 (0.071-0.116)**		**F=3.565; p=0.025**	**CI=0.900; RI=0.933**
6	0.396	0.271 (0.201-0.381)	0.180 (0.121-0.311)	0.124 (0.112-0.130)	0.139 (0.135-0.227)	0.133 (0.120-0.419)		F=4.021; p=0.017	CI=0.900; RI=0.833
7	-0.141	-0.118 ([-0.310]-[-0.026])	-0.158 ([-0.244]-[-0.121])	-0.071 ([-0.161]-[0.054])	-0.189 ([-0.215]-[-0.038])	-0.165 ([-0.197]-[-0.154])		F=1.095; p=0.388	CI=0.692; RI=0.333
8	570.7	891.3 (446.1-1603.3)	733.4 (457.7-3003.4)	2232.1 (1576.0-3384.8)	1451.8 (965.95-2704.2)	999.9 (635.9-1956.8)		F=2.650; p=0.065	CI=0.900; RI=0.800
9	768.9	1110.4 (913.1-1817.9)	886.3 (678.0-1959.3)	1958.7 (1434.5-2248.0)	1523.4 (1132.2-2020.0)	993.0 (630.9-1346.3)		F=3.034; p=0.043	CI=0.750; RI=0.625
10	2161.9	3832.1 (3064.5-5786.3)	2902.1 (1973.9-4222.5)	5080.6 (2318.8-5519.4)	4173.0 (2304.0-5478.5)	3321.8 (749.0-3353.0)		F=1.680; p=0.197	CI=0.750; RI=0.400
11	22.222	0 (0-58.333)	35.000 (13.333-76.667)	28.930 (3.703-55.556)	23.784 (11.111-25.000)	23.333 (0-50.000)	χ^2=361.706; p<0.000		CI=1.000; RI=0/0
12	0	0 (0-45.833)	14.286 (5.000-52.083)	21.935 (1.852-43.377)	3.841 (0-16.667)	20.000 (0-33.333)	χ^2=198.498; p<0.000		CI=0.692; RI=0.667
13	22.222	0 (0-100)	40.000 (0-59.091)	33.333 (20.000-59.090)	50.000 (25.000-83.333)	100 (10.000-100)	χ^2=738.110; p<0.000		CI=0.900; RI=0.500
14	0	0 (0-62.500)	0 (0-20.000)	25.000 (9.524-45.714)	0 (0-4.000)	0	χ^2=100.000; p<0.000		CI=1.000; RI=0/0
15	**2.333**	**3.000 (1.571-9.857)**	**6.250 (4.250-24.000)**	**24.500 (10.333-99.000)**	**11.000 (4.000-29.800)**	**5.800 (3.000-15.500)**	**χ^2=167.534; p<0.000**		**CI=1.000; RI=1.000**
16	1.222	1.667 (1.000-4.714)	2.500 (1.750-9.000)	7.833 (4.200-29.000)	4.000 (2.750-13.600)	2.400 (1.000-3.000)	χ^2=59.613; p<0.000		CI=0.900; RI=0.800

[1] S=siamang, O=orangutan, G=gorilla, C=chimpanzee, B=bonobo, H=human,
[2] Variable identification number
[3] Outgroup data included only in phylogenetic analyses

On the call segment level, tonal structures (variable 3) were found in bonobos and humans, but not in any of the other hominoids (Table 3).

On the call level, call duration (variable 5) and call rhythm (variable 6) showed a tendency of a dichotomy of orangutan-gorilla and chimpanzee-bonobo-human medians and quartiles (Figure 4). However, significant differences were not found for these variables on any taxon dyad (variable 5, Mann-Whitney U tests with Hommel-Hochberg corrections: O-G, O-B, G-B, C-B, C-H, B-H, p>0.05; O-C, p=0.006; O-H, p=0.017; G-C, p=0.016; G-H, p=0.036) (variable 6, Mann-Whitney U tests with Hommel-Hochberg corrections: O-G, G-C, G-B, G-H, C-H; p>0.05; O-C, p=0.01; O-B, p=0.017; O-H, p=0.024; C-B, p=0.016; B-H, p=0.036) (O=orangutan; G=gorilla; C=chimpanzee, B= bonobo; H=human).

On the bout level, medians showed that chimpanzees emitted alternating respiration calls in every fourth bout (variable 14) (Table 3). Humans produced only consecutive exhalation calls. Medians of the remaining hominoid taxa showed less (0%) consecutive exhalation calls per bout. Furthermore, unlike other hominoid medians, orangutan medians indicated less calls (0%) of same rhythm (variable 11), of same call phenotypes (variable 12), and of intervals with <8 milliseconds (variable 13) per bout. The human median of contiguity pattern (variable 13) depicted a high tendency (100%) of call intervals of <8 milliseconds.

On the bout series level, the medians of calls/series (variable 15) of gorillas, chimpanzees, and bonobos, were higher than for humans (Figure 4; Table 3). However, of these three possible taxon dyads, differences were only significant for the chimpanzee-human dyad (Chi-square tests with Hommel-Hochberg corrections: O-G, O-H, G-B, G-H, B-H; p>0.05; O-B, p=0.034; C-B, p=0.023; χ^2=16.809, O-C, p=0.000; χ^2=10.831, G-C, p=0.001; χ^2=11.541, C-H, p=0.001). Since bouts consisted mainly of consecutive exhalation calls (variable 14, see above), this indicated that African apes can emit more consecutive calls in LF tickling bout series than humans.

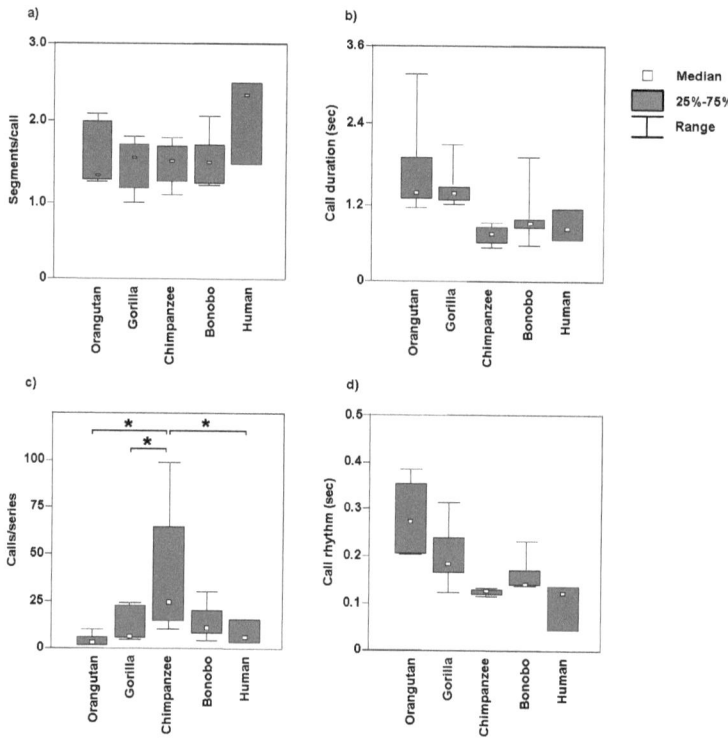

Fig. 4. Medians, quartiles, and ranges of a) segments/call (variable 4), b) call duration (variable 5), c) calls/series (variable 15), and d) call rhythm (variable 6).The first three characters showed strongest support of the exhaustive search tree with CI≥0.900 and RI≥0.900. Significant differences were found only for three taxon dyads of calls/series (Chi-square tests with Hommel-Hochberg corrections: O-G, O-H, G-B, G-H, B-H; p>0.05; O-B, p=0.034; C-B, p=0.023; χ^2=16.809, O-C, p=0.000; χ^2=10.831, G-C, p=0.001; χ^2=11.541, C-H, p=0.001) (O=orangutan; G=gorilla; C=chimpanzee, B= bonobo; H=human). No significant differences were found for any dyads of the remaining variables (see results)

For the remaining variables of all hierarchical sound levels, range values overlapped across all hominoid taxa. Thus, all hominoids showed a more or less comparable taxon variation for all of the hierarchical sound levels measured in LF tickling vocalizations.

Results of Chi-Square tests with Hommel-Hochberg correction indicated significant taxon-specific differences for the 10 nominal acoustic variables (Table 3). One-way ANOVA results with Hommel-Hochberg correction showed no taxon-specific differences for the 6 ordinal acoustic variables.

Phylogenetic analyses of tickling vocalizations

Table 4 depicts the taxon codes of the 16 characters.

Of the 16 characters included in the phylogenetic analysis, three were parsimony-uninformative (Table 3). These were segment tonality (variable 3), rhythm pattern (variable 11), and alternating respiration (variable 14). The remaining 13 characters were parsimony-informative.

Furthermore, data of 3 variables showed highest support of the tree with CI≥0.900 and RI≥0.900. These characters were segments/call (variable 4), call duration (variable 5), and calls/series (variable 15) (Figure 4; Table 3). Of these three variables, significant differences were found only for three taxon dyads of calls/series (see results above). No significant differences were found for any taxon dyads of the other two variables (variable 4, Chi-square tests: O-G, O-C, O-B, O-H, G-C, G-B, G-H, C-B, C-H, B-H; p>0.05) (for variable 5, see results above).

Character state tracings for each of these characters with highest support of the tree are shown in Figure 5. Their results indicated an increase in segments/call, a decrease in call duration, and an increase in calls/series when comparing character states from the root of the cladogram to the chimpanzee-bonobo-human clade. These characters showed changes in temporal complexity.

Table 4. Taxon codes (S, O, G, C, B, H)[1] of the 16 characters. Character states ranged from 0 to 9. The three characters with CI≥0.900 and RI≥0.900 are marked bold.

ID[2]	Sound level & variable	S[3]	O	G	C	B	H
1	Segment noise	9	7	6	7	6	0
2	Segment deterministic chaos	2	0	9	8	9	2
3	Segment tonality	0	0	0	0	0	9
4	**Segments/call**	1	0	2	2	2	9
5	**Call duration**	9	9	9	0	2	1
6	Call rhythm	9	5	2	0	1	0
7	Spectral slope	4	6	2	9	0	2
8	1st spectral moment	0	3	2	9	6	4
9	2nd spectral moment	0	4	1	9	7	2
10	Call peak frequency	0	6	3	9	7	5
11	Rhythm pattern	8	0	9	8	8	8
12	Phenotype pattern	0	0	8	9	5	9
13	Contiguity pattern	6	0	7	7	8	9
14	Alternating respiration	0	0	0	9	0	0
15	**Calls/series**	0	1	3	9	6	3
16	Bouts/series	0	1	3	9	5	2

[1] S=siamang, O=orangutan, G=gorilla, C=chimpanzee, B=bonobo, H=human,
[2] Variable identification number
[3] Outgroup data included only in phylogenetic analyses

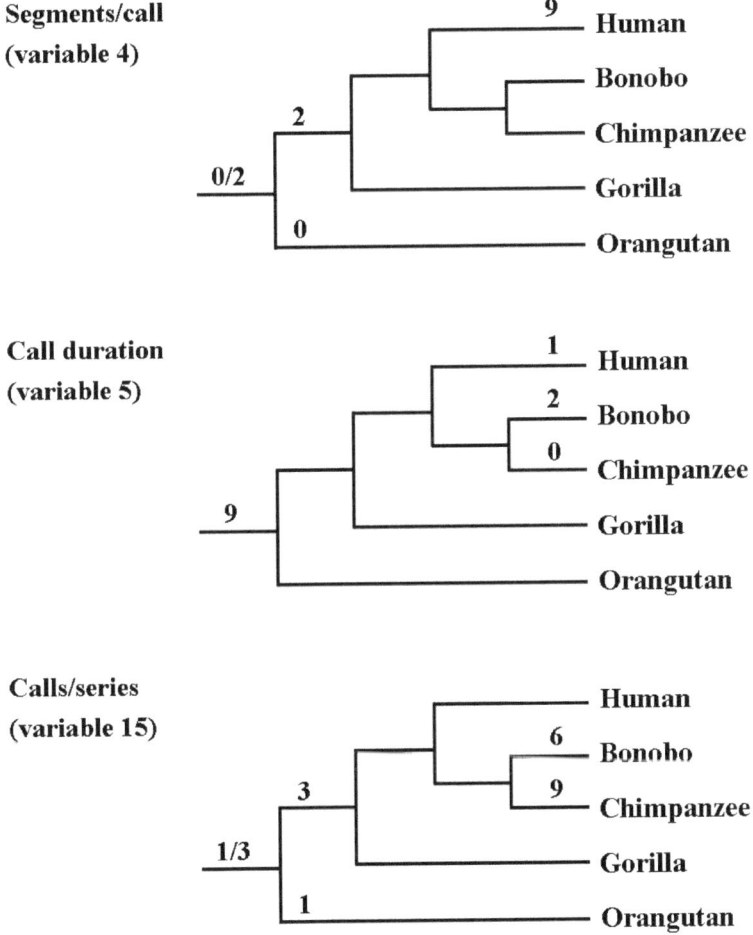

Fig. 5. Character state tracings of individual character evolution for characters with CI≥0.900 and RI≥0.900 of exhaustive search: Segments/call (variable 4), call duration (variable 5), and calls/series (variable 15).

The trees generated by exhaustive search (treelength = 171; CI = 0.8421; RI = 0.6824) and bootstrap analysis with 50% majority-rule are shown in Figure 6. Of the ingroup taxa, the exhaustive search tree depicted chimpanzees and bonobos, as one monophyly, closest to humans. The single orangutan lineage was farthest away from humans. The gorilla lineage took up an intermediary position. Bootstrap results supported all of these monophyletic clades in the exhaustive search tree. Highest bootstrap values were found for the clade of African apes and humans (98) and for the clade of bonobos and chimpanzees (96).

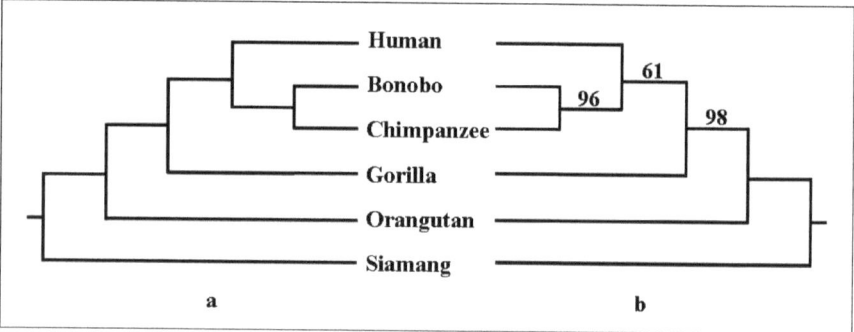

Fig. 6. Two cladograms of 5 hominoid ingroup taxa and siamang as outgroup based on tickling vocalizations: a) Exhaustive search (treelength = 171; CI = 0.8421; RI = 0.6824) and b) bootstrap analysis with 50% majority-rule. Bootstrap values for 1000 replicates are shown above branches.

DISCUSSION

Phylogenetic analyses of this study yielded a topology that clearly split off a single orangutan lineage from the clade of the remaining hominoids. The latter clade, furthermore, depicted a dichotomy with less robustness for the gorilla lineage and chimpanzee-bonobo-human clade. For the latter, there was a robust monophyly of chimpanzees and bonobos. Our resulting tree coincided well with the genetically based topology of hominoids (e.g. McBrearty & Jablongski 2005; Ruvolo et al. 1994; Wildman et al. 2002) (see General Introduction, Figure 5). Thus, phylogenetic results of this study showed that LF tickling vocalizations of great apes and humans are homologous. Consequently, the term vocal laughter seems appropriate for LF tickling vocalizations of great apes.

Thus far, only long distance vocalizations in nonhuman primates were explored for evolutionary perspectives (e.g. Davila Ross & Geissmann 2007; Macedonia & Stanger 1994; Zimmermann 1990). These vocalizations carry species-specific characteristics to communicate over long distances and were found to be inherited in gibbons (Geissmann 1984). For closely related sympatric species, long range calls could be especially important to avoid costs of hybridization (Braune 2006). Since hominoid vocal laughter is soft, our finding demonstrated that phylogenetic reconstructions can also be made based on vocalizations of short distance communication.

Several confounding effects may have altered our acoustic and phylogenetic results. We have included recordings by different recorders who used different equipments. However, recording equipments' frequency responses were flat in the analyzed range. Furthermore, we have downsampled all sounds to 22050 Hz.

Our sample size may appear small. But, it is not easy to obtain high-quality hominoid tickling recordings. In most zoos, tickling sessions by caretakers or experimenters are nowadays not allowed. Also, parent-reared young apes often do not let themselves be tickled by humans. While it is fairly easy to tickle hand-reared young apes, these are rare in zoos. Furthermore, some subjects never vocally laughed when they were tickled.

Age could potentially affect our results due to ontogenetic changes. For instance, human and chimpanzee infants share major commonalities in their vocal system, i.e. a high positioned larynx and its descent relative to the hyoid bone throughout ontogeny (e.g. Lieberman 1984; Lieberman et al. 2001; Nishimura et al. 2003). A low positional larynx yields to more shape diversity of the vocal tract periphery and, therefore, enables individuals to produce more varied and distinct vocalizations as found in speech (Lieberman et al. 1969; Fitch 2000). To minimize potential confounding effects of age on vocal laughter production, we focused in our comparative analysis on infants and young juveniles.

Since body size/mass is known to affect breathing (e.g. Aitken et al. 1986) and formants (reviewed in Fitch 2000), our aim was to reduce possible body size/mass effects on vocal production by focusing on young subjects of comparable age ranges (from 6-12 to 19-56 months).

Moreover, inter-individual variability in vocal laughter may have modified the resolution of the resulting tree. To lessen a possible effect caused by inter-individual variability, taxon medians were used for the phylogenetic analyses. Evidently, despite of such potential effect, a well resolved tree was obtained.

Although all above mentioned factors could influence tickling sound production, it seemed unlikely that they distorted our results since it would have been extremely coincidental if they would have yielded the same topology as known from genetic studies (e.g. Ruvolo et al. 1994).

Results of character state tracings of the three characters most supportive of our topology revealed that throughout hominoid evolution the number of segments per call and the number of calls per series increased and the call duration decreased. These findings suggested a general increase in temporal complexity of vocal laughter, that reached its peak prior to the last common ancestor of chimpanzees, bonobos, and humans, but after their separation from the gorillas. Such growth in temporal complexity most likely marks an integral period in hominoid vocal laughter evolution. It could reflect evolutionary changes in its vocal production due to function (see chapter 1) and breathing systems (MacLarnon & Hewitt 1999, 2004). However, since vocal production is also affected by vocal capacities and controls (e.g. Fitch et al. 2002; Jürgens 2002a, b; Owren et al. 1997), these factors could have influenced such phylogenetic modifications.

This study provided evidence that all hominoids emit vocal laughter calls which can have energy distributions of either noise or deterministic chaos. Taken together, our findings and those by Vettin and Todt (2005) suggested that tonal laughter is present in chimpanzees, bonobos, and humans --- the three taxa that were found in this study to emit vocal laughter of highest temporal complexity. The lack of tonal structures in vocal laughter of orangutans and gorillas and its presence in the remaining hominoids may be explained by differences in function and/or its effect on listeners. Interestingly, unvoiced (i.e. atonal) human vocal laughter is perceived as less positive than voiced (i.e. tonal) human vocal laughter by listeners (Bachorowski & Owren 2001). Alternatively, differences in vocal laughter between these taxa may be due to different vocal capacities and/or vocal control.

Another major difference between results of Vettin and Todt's (2005) study and this study lies in the presence of alternating respiratory calls. While Vettin and Todt (2005) reported that chimpanzee vocal laughter consisted mostly of alternating expiration-inspiration calls, we found that such calls were only present in every fourth bout of our chimpanzee subjects and were even less frequent in the other great apes. All other bouts consisted of consecutive expiration calls. These findings strongly contradicted Provine's (1996) postulation that great apes are incapable of emitting consecutive exhalation calls during vocal laughter and that this limit mirrors their incapability to speak. Our data even showed that all African apes can produce more consecutive exhalation calls per bout series than humans. The largest number of consecutive exhalation calls we found was emitted by a bonobo with 65 calls (data of this study). It seems unlikely that bout series of more than 10-20 consecutive exhalation calls are produced without inhalations. Thus, we assumed that African apes are able to inhale during vocal laughter bout series without intervening much with the rhythmical pattern of laughter. Furthermore, we predicted that African apes can extend their exhalation phases during vocal laughter, similar to humans (e.g. Provine 2004). Such control of breathing while vocalizing mirrors the mechanisms applied by humans during speech (e.g. Winkworth et al. 1995; MacLarnon & Hewitt 1999). This way, our results contradicted MacLarnon and Hewitt's (1999) postulation that humans can expand their exhalation phases while vocalizing more than nonhuman primates and that such an improved breathing control in humans gave a leeway to the evolution of speech.

To sum up, this study provided first empirical evidence for a pre-human basis of human vocal laughter. As shown by character state tracings, an clear phylogenetic change in the evolution of hominoid vocal laughter involved its increase in temporal complexity, which emerged after the gorilla lineage branched off the chimpanzee-bonobo-human clade but prior to the separation of the latter. Within the same time window, tonal properties in hominoid vocal laughter must have evolved. Most likely, these phylogenetic changes of hominoid vocal laughter production were coupled by modifications in function, breathing systems, and/or vocal capacities and controls.

ACKNOWLEDGMENTS

We are very grateful to S. Nathan, P. Andau, E. Bosi, and H. Bernard for their logistic help at Sepilok Orangutan Rehabilitation Centre, to M. Wessels and R. Shockley for their assistance in the recording collection, to S. Menzler for her statistical advice, and to R. Brüning for technical support. Furthermore, we profited from the discussion with members of the DFG FOR-499. The data collection was carried out in Sepilok Orangutan Rehabilitation Centre, Apenheul Primate Park (Apeldoorn), Zoo Wilhelma (Stuttgart), Schwaben Park (Kaiserbach), Zoologischer Garten Berlin, Zoo Frankfurt, Zoo Hannover, Zoo Wuppertal, and in the homes of Faidi, Im, and Bartz. This study was funded by University of Veterinary Medicine Hannover, Center for Systems Neuroscience, Forschungszentrum Jülich GmbH, and Freundeskreis der Tierärztlichen Hochschule Hannover e.V. The field study was approved by Sabah Wildlife Department and Economic Planning Unit, Malaysia.

REFERENCES

Aitken, M. L., Franklin, J. L., Pierson, D. J., & Schoene, R. B. 1986 Influence of body size and gender on control of ventilation. J. Appl. Physiol. 60, 1894-1899.

Archangelsky, M. 2004 Higher-level phylogeny of Hydrophilinae (Coleoptera: Hydrophilidae) based on larval, pupal and adult characters. Syst. Entomol. 29, 188-214.

Bachorowski, J.-A. & Owren, M.J. 2001 Not all laughs are alike: Voiced but not unvoiced laughter readily elicits positive affect. Psych. Science 12 (3), 252-257.

Baldwin, J.D. & Baldwin, J.I. 1976 Vocalizations of howler monkeys (*Alouatta palliata*) in Southwestern Panama. Folia Primatol. 26, 81-108.

Bekoff, M. & Byers, J.A. 1981 A crytical reanalysis of the ontogeny and phylogeny of mammalian social and locomotor play: an ethological hornet's nest. In Behavioral development (eds. K. Immelmann, G. Barlow, M. Main, & L. Petrinovich), pp. 296-337. Cambridge: Cambridge University Press.

Bekoff, M. 1995 Play signals as punctuation: the structure of social play in canids. Behaviour 132 (5-6), 419-429.

Biben, M. 1998 Squirrel monkey play fighting: making the case for a cognitive training function for play. In Animal play: Evolutionary, comparative, and ecological perspectives (eds. M. Bekoff & J.A. Byers), pp. 161-182. Cambridge: Cambridge University Press.

Boersma, P. & Weenink, D. 2007. Praat: doing phonetics by computer (Version 4.5.16) [Computer program]. Retrieved February 18.

Braune,P. 2006 Acoustic variability and its biological significance in noctural lemurs, Hannover: Universität Hannover, 100 p.

Chevalier-Skolnikoff, S. 1982 A cognitive analysis of facial behavior in Old World monkeys, apes, and human beings. Primate communication, (eds. C.T. Snowdon, C.H. Brown, & M.R. Petersen), pp. 303-368. Cambridge: Cambridge University Press.

Cleveland, J. & Snowdon, C.T. 1982 The complex vocal repertoire of the adult cotton-top tamarin (*Saguinus oedipus oedipus*). Z. Tierpsychol. 58, 231-270.

Davila Ross, M. & Geissmann, T. 2007 Call diversity of wild male orangutans: A phylogenetic approach. Am. J. Primatol. 69, 305-324.

de Waal, F.B.M. 1988 The communicative repertoire of captive bonobos (*Pan paniscus*) compared to that of chimpanzees. Behaviour 106, 183-251.

Eibl-Eibesfeldt, I. 1985 Der vorprogrammierte Mensch. Kiel: Orion-Heimreiter-Verlag.

Ekman, P. 1973 Cross-cultural studies of facial expression. In Darwin and facial expression (ed. P. Ekman), pp. 169–222. New York: Academic Press.

Eriksson, E.J., Cepeda, L.F., Rodman, R.D., McAlister, D.F., Bitzer, D., & Arroway, P. 2004 Cross-language speaker identification using spectral moments. Fonetik, Dept. of Linguistics, Stockholm University.

Fagan, R.M. 1981 Animal play behavior. New York: Oxford University Press.

Farris, J. 1989. The retention index and the resealed consistency index. Cladistics 5, 417-419.

Felsenstein, J. 1985 Confidence limits on phylogenies: An approach using the bootstrap. Evolution 39 (4), 783-791.

Fischer, J., Hammerschmidt, K., Cheney, D.L., Seyfarth, R.M. 2001 Acoustic features of female chacma baboon barks. Ethology 107(1), 33-54.

Fitch, W.T. 2000 The evolution of speech: a comparative review. Trends Cognit. Sci. 4, 258-267.

Fitch, W.T., Neubauer, J., & Herzel, H. 2002 Calls out of chaos: the adaptive significance of nonlinear phenomena in mammalian vocal production. Anim. Behav. 63, 407-418.

Förderreuther, B. & Zimmermann, E. 2003 "Laughter" in bonobos?: Preliminary results of an acoustic analysis of tickling sounds in a hand-reared male. Folia Primatol. 74, 193-194.

Fossey, D. 1983 Gorillas in the mist. Boston: Houghton Mifflin.

Freedman, J.L. & Perlick, D. 1979 Crowding, contagion, and laughter. J. Exp. Soc. Psychol. 15, 295-303.

Garcia-Cruz, J. & Sosa, V. 2006 Coding quantitative character data for phylogenetic analysis: A comparison of five methods. Syst. Botany 31(2), 302-309.

Geissmann, T. 1984 Inheritance of song parameters in the gibbon song, analysed in 2 hybrid gibbons (*Hylobates pileatus* x *H. lar*). Folia Primatol. 42, 216-235.

Gervais, M., Wilson, D.S. 2005 The evolution and functions of laughter and humor: a synthetic approach. Quart. Rev. Biol. 80, 395-430.

Goodall, J. 1986 The chimpanzees of Gombe: Patterns of behavior. Cambridge: Harvard University Press.

Harris, C. 1999 The mystery of ticklish laughter. Am. Sci. 87(4), 344-350.

Hochberg, Y. & Hommel, G. 1998 Step-up multiple testing procedures. Encyclopedia Statist. Sci. (Supp.) 2.

Jürgens, U. 2002a A study of the central control of vocalization using the squirrel monkey. Med. Eng. Phys. 24, 473-477.

Jürgens, U. 2002b Neural pathways underlying vocal control. Neurosci. Biobehav. Rev. 26, 235-258.

Kitching, I.J., Forey, P.L., Humphries, C.J., & Williams, D.M. 1998 Cladistics: The theory and practice of parsimony analysis. New York: Oxford University Press. xiii+228 p.

Lieberman, P., Klatt, D. H., & Wilson, W. H. 1969 Vocal tract limitations on the vowel repertoires of rhesus monkeys and other nonhuman primates. Science 164, 1185-1187.

Lieberman, D.E. 1984 The biology and evolution of language. Cambridge: Harvard University Press.

Lieberman, D.E., McCarthy, R.C., Hiiemae, K.M. & Palmer, J.B. 2001 Ontogeny of postnatal hyoid and larynx descent in humans. Arch. Oral Biol. 46, 117-128.

Locke, J.L., Bekken, K.E., McMinn-Larson, L. & Wein, D. 1995 Emergent control of manual and vocal-motor activity in relation to the development of speech. Brain Lang. 51, 498-508.

Macedonia J.M. & Stanger K.F. 1994. Phylogeny of the Lemuridae revisited: Evidence from communication signals. Folia Primatol. 63, 1-43.

MacLarnon, A. & Hewitt, G. 2004 Increased breathing control: Another factor in the evolution of human language. Evol. Anthropol. 13:181-197.

MacLarnon, A.M. & Hewitt, G.P. 1999 The evolution of human speech: the role of enhanced breathing control. Am. J. Phys. Anthropol. 109:341-363.

Maddison, D.R. & Maddison, W.P. 2000. MacClade 4: Analysis of phylogeny and character evolution. Sunderland, Massachusetts: Sinauer Associates. 492 p.

Marshall, A.J., Wrangham, R.W., & Arcadi, A.C. 1999. Does learning affect the structure of vocalizations in chimpanzees? Anim. Behav. 58, 825-830.

McBrearty,S. & Jablonski, N.G. First fossil chimpamzee. Nature 437 (1.9.), 105-108, 2005.

Nishimura, T., Mikami, A., Suzuki, J., & Matsuzawa, T. 2003 Descent of the larynx in chimpanzee infants. Proc.Natl.Acad.Sci.U.S.A. 100 (12):6930-6933.

Owren, M.J., Seyfarth, R.M., & Cheney, D.L. 1997. The acoustic features of vowel-like grunt calls in chacma baboons (*Papio cynocephalus ursinus*): Implications for production processes and functions. J. Acoust. Soc. Am., 101, 2951-2963.

Panksepp, J. & Burgdorf, J. 2003 "Laughing" rats and the evolutionary antecedents of human joy? Physiol. Behav. 79, 533-547.

Patterson, C. 1988 Homology in classical and molecular biology. Mol. Biol Evol. 5(6), 603-625.

Provine, R.R. 1996 Laughter. Am. Sci. 84, 38-45.

Provine, R.R. 2004 Laughing, tickling, and the evolution of speech and self. Curr. Direct. Psychol. Sci. 13 (6), 215-218.

Riede, T., Wilden, I., & Tembrock, G. 1997 Subharmonics, biphonations, and frequency jumps - common components of mammalian vocalization or indicators for disorders? Z Säugetier 62 (Suppl 2):198–203.

Riede, T., Owren, M.J., & Arcadi, A.C. 2004 Nonlinear acoustics in pant hoots of common chimpanzees (*Pan troglodytes*): Frequency jumps, subharmonics, biphonation, and deterministic chaos. Am. J. Primatol. 64, 277–291.

Rijksen, H.D. 1978. A fieldstudy on Sumatran orang utans (*Pongo pygmaeus abelii*, Lesson 1827). Ecology, behaviour and conservation. Wageningen: Veenman H, Zones BV.

Robillard, T., Höbel, G. & Gerhardt, H.C. 2006 Evolution of advertising signals in North American hylid frogs: Vocalizations as end-products of calling behavior. Cladistics 22, 1-13.

Robins, R.L. & McCreery, E.K. 2003 African wild dog pup vocalizations with special reference to Morton's Model. Behaviour 140, 333-351.

Rodman, R., McAllister, D., Bitzer, D. Cepeda, L., & Abbit, P. 2002 Forensic speaker identification based on spectral moments. Forensic Linguistics 9(1), 1350-1771.

Ruvolo, M., Pan, D., Zehr, S., Goldberg, T., Disotell, T.R. & von Dornum, M. 1994 Gene trees and hominoid phylogeny. Proc. Natl. Acad. Sci. USA. 91, 8900-8904.

Scheiner, E., Hammerschmidt, K., Jürgens, U. & Zwirner, P. 2002 Acoustic analyses of developmental changes and emotional expression in the preverbal vocalizations of infants. J. Voice 16 (4), 509-529.

Schenkel, R. 1964 Zur Ontogenese des Verhaltens bei Gorilla und Mensch. Zeitschrift Morphologie und Anthropologie. 54, 233-259

Sroufe, L.A. & Wunsch, J.P. 1972 The development of laughter in the first year of life. Child Devel. 43, 1326-1344.

Struhsaker, T.T. 1975 The red colobus monkey. Chicago: University of Chicago Press.

Swofford, D.L. 1990, PAUP: Phylogenetic analysis using parsimony. Campaign, Illinois: Computer program distributed by Illinois Natural History Survey (3).

Tabachnick, B.G. & Fidell, L.S. 2007 Using multivariate statistics, Boston: Pearson Education, Inc.

Taglialatela, J.P., Savage-Rumbaugh, E.S., & Baker, L.A. 2003 Vocal production by a language competent *Pan paniscus*. Int. J. Primatol. 24 (1).

Thiele, K. 1993 The holy grail of the perfect character: The cladistic treatment of morphometric data. Cladistics 9, 275-304.

Tokuda, I., Riede,T., Neubauer, J., Owren, M.J., & Herzel, H-P. 2002 Nonlinear analysis of irregular animal vocalizations. J. Acoust. Soc. Am. 111, 2908-2919.

Preuschoft, S. 1995 'Laughter' and 'smiling' in macaques - an evolutionary perspective. Utrecht: Rijksuniversiteit, 254 p.

van Hooff, J.A.R.A.M. & Preuschoft, S. 2003 Laughter and smiling: The intertwining of nature and culture. In Animal social complexity: Intelligence, culture, and individualized societies (eds F.B.M. de Waal & P.L. Tyack), pp 261-287. Cambridge: Harvard University Press.

van Hooff, J.A.R.A.M. 1972 A comparative approach to the phylogeny of laughter and smiling. Non-verbal communication (ed. R. A. Hinde), pp. 209-241. Cambridge: Cambridge University Press.

Vettın, J. & Todt, D. 2004 Laughter in conversation: Features of occurrence and acoustic structure. J. Nonverb. Behav. 28 (2), 93-115.

Vettin, J. & Todt, D. 2005 Human laughter, social play, and play vocalizations of non-human primates: an evolutionary approach. Behaviour 142, 217-240.

Wildman, D.E., Grossman, L.I., & Goodman, M. 2002 Functional DNA in humans and chimpanzees shows that they are more similar to each other than either is to other apes. Probing human origins (eds. M. Goodman, A.S. Moffat), pp. 1-10. Cambridge: American Academy of Arts and Sciences.

Winkworth, A.L., Davis, P.J., Adams, [2] R.D., Ellis, E. 1995 Breathing patterns during spontaneous speech. J. Speech Hear. Res. 38. 124-144.

Zimmermann, E. 1989 Aspects of reproduction and behavioral and vocal development in Senegal bushbabies (*Galago senegalensis*). Int. J. Primatol. 10 (1), 1-17.

Zimmermann, E. 1990 Differentiation of vocalizations in bushbabies (Galaginae, Prosimiae, Primates) and the significance for assessing phylogenetic relationships. Z Zool Syst Evol-forschg 28, 217-239.

Zimmermann, E. 1991 Ontogeny of acoustic communication in prosimian primates. Primatology today (eds. A. Ehara, O. Takenaka, & M. Iwamoto), pp. 337-340. Amsterdam: Elsevier.

Zimmermann, E. 1995 Loud calls in nocturnal prosimians: structure, evolution and ontogeny. Current topics in primate vocal communication (eds. E. Zimmermann, J. D. Newman, & U. Jürgens) p. 47-72, New York: Plenum Press.

GENERAL DISCUSSION

VOCAL LAUGHTER PHYLOGENY

In Chapter 3, I assessed the phylogenetic relationship of great ape low-frequency (LF) vocalizations and human vocal laughter during tickling sessions. The resulting cladogram showed a first split off for the orangutan lineage followed by a split off for the gorilla lineage. Within the monophyly of chimpanzee-bonobo-human, a dichotomy of chimpanzee-bonobo and man was depicted. This phylogenetic tree coincided with the topology widely accepted in systematics based on genetic studies (e.g. McBrearty & Jablongski 2005; Ruvolo et al. 1994; Wildman et al. 2002) (also see General Introduction, Figure 5). Due to these results, I concluded that LF tickling vocalizations of great apes and human vocal laughter share the same phylogenetic origin. Thus, I used the term vocal laughter to further describe these great ape vocalizations.

TICKLING AND SOCIAL PLAY

Embedded in the General Introduction, the extent to which facial displays are exhibited by great apes when they vocally laugh during tickling sessions was assessed. I focused on the phylogenetically most distanced great apes, the orangutan, and found that this species regularly emitted open-mouth faces (e.g. ROM displays and OMBT displays), tickling bites, and nonrelaxed faces while vocally laughing (see General Introduction, Table 3; also see Chapter 2, Table 1 for definitions on facial displays). Our results demonstrated that vocal laughter of great apes is not strictly linked to the occurrence of specific facial displays themselves. In addition, it is important to note, that orangutans emit the same facial displays during tickling session as during social play (Davila Ross pers. obs.), that tickling is a component of social play in great apes (e.g. Fossey 1983; Goodall 1986), and that vocal laughter of tickling sessions are perceived by human listeners as the same as LF vocalization of social play (e.g. Davila Ross pers. obs.; Vettin & Todt 2005). Based on these findings, I concluded that vocal laughter of great apes evoked during tickling sessions is homologous to the LF vocalizations in social play. Therefore, I used the term vocal laughter for LF vocalizations of both sound-releasing contexts.

THE FUNCTION OF ORANGUTAN VOCAL LAUGHTER

In Chapter 1, I evaluated the function of orangutan vocal laughter for the following three hypotheses on the emergence of hominoid laughter: 1) Vocal laughter as an expression of high arousal/thrill activates playmates to continue with play (to test the Play activation hypothesis); 2) older playmates, who incorporate more danger to the younger playmate than vice versa, vocally laugh more often than younger playmates to signal that there is no danger of play to escalate into real aggression (to test the Non-aggression hypothesis); and 3) younger playmates vocally laugh more often than older playmates to appease the play situation in order to protect themselves from getting injured (to test the Protection hypothesis). Our results showed that orangutan vocal laughter was neither used more often by older nor younger playmates. Thus, the Non-aggression and Protection hypotheses were rejected. Furthermore, our data showed tendencies that both playmates prolong their play actions and depicted that entire play bouts lasted longer. This supported the Play activation hypothesis. Therefore, this study showed that, orangutans emit vocal laughter as an expression of arousal/thrill, which activates playmates to maintain play. Since such function of play panting (i.e. vocal laughter) was also found in chimpanzees (Matsusaka 2004), our finding suggested phylogenetic continuity in vocal laughter function across hominoids.

FACIAL MIMICRY IN SOCIAL PLAY OF ORANGUTANS

One of the properties that add to the phenomenology of human laughter is its contagion (Lundqvist 1995; Provine 1992). Since human facial displays convey emotions (e.g. Ekman 2003) and since emotions can be perceived by others, e.g. by means of facial congruency (e.g. Hatfield et al. 1994), I found it likely that such mechanisms of behavioral congruency of man exist in nonhuman primates. Thus, I tested in Chapter 2 if orangutans rapidly (≤1 second) mimic open-mouth faces (e.g. ROM displays and OMBT displays) of their conspecifics in social play (see Chapter 2, Table 1 for definitions on facial displays). Our statistic approach was constructed to exclude possible confounding effects of specific playmate constellations, play contexts, play intensities, the presence of physical contact, and play bites by standardizing the compared scenes of this study. In addition, no vocalizations were produced during the scenes that were evaluated. This study showed that orangutans rapidly emit open-mouth faces after seeing open-mouth faces in their playmates. This suggested that, like humans for the facial expression of laughter (e.g. Dimberg & Thunberg 1998), great apes may show open-mouth face contagion. Interestingly, this study showed that experience plays an integral role in the presence of rapid facial mimicry, since I found this mechanism present in juveniles and subadults, but not in infants.

THE EVOLUTION OF THE OPEN-MOUTH BARED-TEETH DISPLAY

Because the ROM display is found in New World monkeys, prosimians, and canids, and is, together with the OMBT display, common in Old World monkeys, it seems likely that this expression is ancestral to the OMBT display. (reviewed in van Hooff & Preuschoft 2003). Yet, what phylogenetic pattern these displays show across great apes was still nebulous.

Throughout our studies, the ROM display and OMBT display were observed in all great apes during tickling sessions and play (Davila Ross pers. obs.). These findings can fill the gaps of knowledge on the usage of these displays in great apes --- specifically, orangutans and gorillas. I found that orangutans exhibit OMBT displays clearly more often than ROM displays (Davila Ross pers. obs.). Thus far, these facial displays of orangutans were only briefly commented on (e.g. Chevalier-Skolnikoff 1982). Much less was even known about gorillas. I found that gorillas regularly exhibit ROM and OMBT displays (Davila Ross unpubl. data).

The usage of these displays was already well known for chimpanzees and bonobos. Interestingly, although chimpanzees are commonly known for their frequently occurring ROM displays (e.g. Flack et al. 2004; Waller & Dunbar 2005), full play faces (i.e. OMBT displays) may range from being absent (van Hooff 1972) to being as frequently present as play faces (i.e. ROM displays) (see Palagi 2006, Figure 4). Bonobos are known for emitting full play faces (i.e. OMBT displays) more frequently than play faces (i.e. ROM displays) (e.g. Palagi 2006). All these findings suggested phylogenetic continuity of the ROM and OMBT displays in great apes (see Table 1 for overview).

Thus, the OMBT display is not only present in many Old World monkeys, but also in all great apes. Although there certainly may be socio-ecological factors affecting the occurrence of the OMBT display in primates, as suggested by Preuschoft (1995), I found that the OMBT display, like the ROM display, evidently shows phylogenetic continuity in its appearance in primate evolution. Therefore, I predicted that the OMBT display fully evolved within the time window between the emergence of Old World monkeys and the emergence of great apes (see Figure 1 for scheme). Due to its contextual (Preuschoft 1995) and morphological (see General Introduction, Table 1 for morphological characteristics) closeness to the ROM display and their occurrence with vocal laughter, I hypothesized that the OMBT display originated from the ROM display (see Figure 1).

Table 1. Overview of the occurrence of the relaxed open-mouth (i.e. ROM) display and the open-mouth bared-teeth (i.e. OMBT) display in great apes during social play and tickling.

Taxon	Social play		Tickling	
	ROM display	OMBT display	ROM display	OMBT display
Orangutans	See Chapter 2, Table 1	see Chapter 2, Table 1	See General Introduction, Table 3	See General Introduction, Table 3
Gorillas	Davila Ross pers. obs.	Davila Ross pers. obs.	Davila Ross pers. obs.	Davila Ross pers. obs.
Chimpanzees	e.g. van Hooff 1972	e.g. Palagi 2006*	e.g. van Hooff 1972	Davila Ross pers. obs.
Bonobos	e.g. Palagi 2006*	e.g. de Waal 1988	Davila Ross pers. obs.	Davila Ross pers. obs.

*=full play face

The ROM display and the OMBT display both differ in the degree of baring teeth. Whereas the OMBT display shows upper as well as lower tooth rows, the ROM display shows only the lower tooth row (see General Introduction, Table 1 for morphological characteristics). However, by baring the upper tooth row, the OMBT display seems close to identical to the Duchenne laughter.

Since there are morphological similarities of the nonhuman primate OMBT display with the human Duchenne laughter and since the OMBT display, like the ROM display, can accompany hominoid vocal laughter (e.g. van Hooff & Preuschoft 2003) and frequently occurs in hominoid social play (see Table 1; also see above), I hypothesized that the nonhuman primate OMBT display and the human Duchenne laughter are the identical manifestation (see Figure 1 for scheme). Thus, I find the term "facial laughter" appropriate to describe the OMBT display.

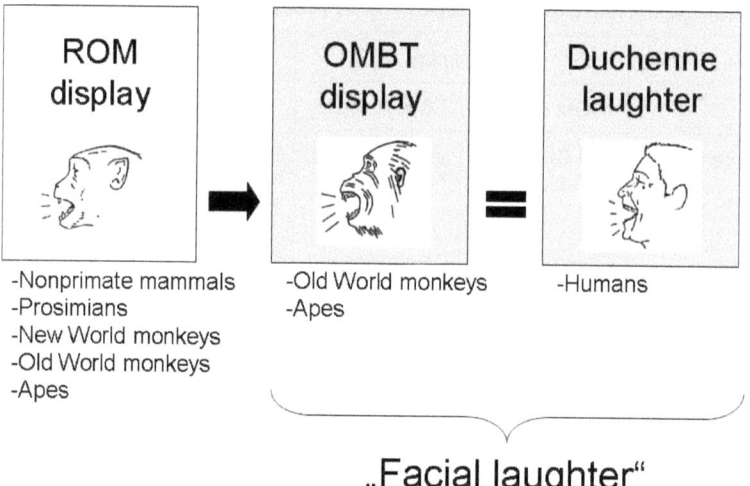

Figure 1. Proposed scheme of "facial laughter" evolution. The relaxed open-mouth (i.e. ROM) display is ancestral to both the open-mouth bared-teeth (i.e. OMBT) display and Duchenne laughter. I postulated that the OMBT display of nonhuman primates and Duchenne laughter of humans are the identical manifestation and, therefore, used the term "facial laughter" for this display. Furthermore, I found it likely that facial laughter evolved from the ROM display after the emergence of Old World monkeys but prior to the emergence of hominoids. Drawings were partially adapted from van Hooff (1972).

THE ROLE OF THE OMBT DISPLAY IN THE EVOLUTION OF "SMILE" AND "LAUGHTER"

In 1972, van Hooff proposed that the SBT display with its similarity in morphological characteristics and contexts embodies the nonhuman primate homologous mode of human smile. Hereby, he characterized three types of silent bared-teeth (SBT) displays in chimpanzees as horizontal, vertical, and open-mouth SBT displays (see General Introduction, Figure 3).

It is important to note that, van Hooff (1972) implied that the chimpanzee "open-mouth SBT" display, which is a silent expression of affinitive behavior, is morphologically closer to the human Duchenne laughter than the ROM display. Because of this and because the ROM display occurs in play and is often accompanied by staccato breathing (i.e. vocal laughter) (see above), he postulated that the SBT display converged with the ROM display as one manifestation of playful context to ritualize as the facial expression of laughter in *Homo* (see General Introduction, Figure 3 for the phylogenetic development suggested by van Hooff 1972).

However, in our view, the chimpanzee "open-mouth SBT" display of van Hooff's (1972) study is morphologically equivalent to the chimpanzee OMBT display (compare General Introduction, Figure 3, to General Introduction, Table 1, for morphological characteristics of "open-mouth SBT" and OMBT displays, respectively). As their names already indicate, both are expressions of open-mouths and bared-teeth.

A notable difference between these two displays lies in the contexts in which they appear. While displays of open-mouths and bared-teeth occurred only in affinitive contexts, not in play, in van Hooff's (1972) chimpanzees, such displays were found in social play of other chimpanzee colonies (e.g. Goodall 1986; Palagi 2006). Interestingly, the study of Preuschoft (1995) has demonstrated that socio-ecological factors can affect the presence of the OMBT displays in behavioral contexts of closely related species. Moreover, she suggested that they may also influence across human cultures. For instance, laughter may be more inhibited in cultures of a more despotic social organization than laughter of a more egalitarian social organization. Furthermore, chapter 2 has demonstrated that experience affects the usage of ROM and OMBT displays in facial mimicry during orangutan play. Similarly, the occurrence of play faces (i.e. ROM displays) may depend on the presence of other individuals close by (Flack et al. 2004). Based on these findings, I proposed that a nonhuman primate group may use the OMBT display differently than another colony of the same species based on differences in their social environment.

Another difference between the "open-mouth SBT" display and the OMBT display lies in the presence of vocal laughter. While OMBT displays of great apes can be accompanied by "panting laughs" (i.e. vocal laughter) (e.g. de Waal 1988), the "open-mouth SBT" displays of van Hooff's (1972) study were silent. However, since great ape vocal laughter is likely to be an expression of thrill/arousal that activates playmates to continue with play (Matsusaka 2004; also see Chapter 1), vocal laughter should not be expected for an affinitive contexts of the OMBT display (van Hooff 1972).

Therefore, I considered the "open-mouth SBT" display of chimpanzees in van Hooff's (1972) study and the OMBT display as one and the same manifestation, namely the OMBT display.

Since, there is evidence that the OMBT display evolved from the ROM display (see above), van Hooff's (1972) postulation on the evolution of "smile" and "laughter" needs to be reconsidered. If the "open-mouth SBT" display of chimpanzees in van

Hooff's (1972) study is omitted from his proposed scheme exhibited for the emergence of laughter, then there is not much hold that the Duchenne laughter in any part emerged from smile (see General Introduction, Figure 3 for the phylogenetic development suggested by van Hooff 1972).

Thus, I hypothesized there was no morphological convergence of the SBT display and facial laughter that ritualized to the Duchenne laughter and that the human Duchenne laughter is identical to the nonhuman primate OMBT display.

SUMMING IT UP

Our results showed phylogenetic continuity in function and usage of hominoid vocal and facial laughter, respectively (see Table 2 for an overview on outcomes of our study). Although there seem to be socio-ecological factors influencing the presence of the OMBT display, it is present across all great ape species and in humans. Furthermore, I have found that all great apes and humans emit vocal laughter. Interestingly, despite all these commonalities, taxon-specific differences were evident in the acoustic production. Our study hinted that there was a phylogenetic change after the separation of *Gorilla* from *Pan* and *Homo*, but before the taxa of the latter clade branched off. The acoustic changes implied increase in spectral and temporal complexity. Furthermore, vocal laughter seemed to increase in amplitude and in number of occurrences from *Pongo* to *Pan* and *Homo*. It would be interesting to find out if vocal laughter of *Pan* and *Homo* with such acoustic cues evokes different responses in conspecifics than vocal laughter without these acoustic cues. These findings suggested that vocal laughter became more important along this phylogenetic road, despite showing little changes in facial morphology, facial mimicry, and vocal function.

Table 2. Overview of facial morphology, facial mimicry, bioacoustics, and vocal function of facial and vocal laughter in macaques (*Macaca* spp.), orangutans (*Pongo* spp.), gorillas (*Gorilla* spp.), chimpanzees/bonobos (*Pan* spp.), and humans (*Homo* spp.). Drawings were partially adapted from van Hooff (1972).

	Facial morphology	Facial mimicry	Bioacoustics	Vocal function
Macaca spp.	OMBT display	?	?	
Pongo spp.		Facial mimicry	— Atonal laughter	To maintain play
Gorilla spp.	h h OMBT display	?		?
Pan spp.			— Origin of tonal laughter	To maintain play
Homo spp.	ha ha Duchenne laughter	Facial mimicry	— Increase of temporal complexity	To maintain play

Altogether, this thesis provided evidence on phylogenetic continuity of human and great ape laughter for their facial and vocal manifestations in morphological characteristics, function, and phenomenology. Therefore, it demonstrated that laughter must have evolved at least 12-16 million years ago (Goodman et al. 1998).

GENERAL ACKNOWLEDGMENTS

I am most grateful to my supervisor, Prof. Elke Zimmermann, for her wonderful guidance and her strong commitment throughout this study. She has been an invaluable mentor and an inspiration throughout this time. Furthermore, I would like to thank my co-supervisors Prof. Eckart Altenmüller and Prof. Reinhard Dengler for their guidance. Many thanks go to Prof. Uwe Jürgens who agreed to become the external reviewer of my thesis. Thank you all for your commitment and time on the evaluation of this thesis.

Special thanks go to Michael J. Owren, who advised me on the acoustic analysis of this thesis. I am also much obliged to Birgit Förderreuther, whose recordings immensely improved the data collection of the acoustic study. Many thanks go to Susanne Menzler and Ute Radespiel for their statistical advice and to Rüdiger Brüning and Luis Pauchard for technical support.

I am very grateful for having had the opportunity to conduct this thesis. Such was made possible by the University of Veterinary Medicine Hannover and by my PhD-program Center for Systems Neuroscience Hannover. Particularly, I would like to thank hereby Prof. W. Baumgärtner, Dr. D. Esser, Dr. S. Schwab, Mrs. N. Borsum, and Mrs. K. Stark.

Many thanks go to M. Wessels, B. Tia, P. Hristozova, C. Schopf, R. Shockley, R. Malkus, E. Ey, K. Jochum, and L.-M. Gerhardt for their assistance and to The RISE-program of the DAAD which opened doors for apprenticeships. Also I would like to thank E. Engelke for her help in the videometric analysis.

I profited from the discussions with members of DFG FOR-499 and the graduate students of Perspectives of Primatology, German Primate Center.

The data collection was carried out with the support of Sepilok Orangutan Rehabilitation Centre (SORC), Zoo Wilhelma (Stuttgart), Schwaben Park (Kaiserbach), Zoologischer Garten Berlin, Zoo Hannover, Tierpark Hagenbeck Hamburg, Apenheul Primate Park (Apeldoorn), Zoo Leipzig, MPI for Evolutionary Anthropology, Zoo Münster, Serengeti-Park Hodenhagen, Zoo Frankfurt, and Zoo Wuppertal. Hereby would like to especially thank Dr. S. Nathan, Dr. P. Andau, Dr. E. Bosi, Dr. H. Bernard, S. Alsisto, Dr. H. Engel, K. Meyer, Prof. M. Böer, R. Schirsching, Dr. M. Holtkötter, E. Kastner, Dr. P. Rahn, R Opitz, R. Gralki, Dr. F. Rietkerk, Prof. M. Tomasello, D. Hanus, B. Uphoff, Dr. D. Encke, Dr. T. Knauf, and Dr. K. Wermke. Many thanks to the families Faidi, Im, and Bartz for the human laughter recordings.

Research was funded by University of Veterinary Medicine Hannover, Center for Systems Neuroscience, Forschungszentrum Jülich GmbH, Frauenförderung der Stiftung Tierärztliche Hochschule Hannover, and Freundeskreis der Tierärztlichen Hochschule Hannover e.V. The field study in SORC was approved by Sabah Wildlife Department and Economic Planning Unit, Malaysia.

I would like to thank most dearly my parents, Jose and Burglind Dávila, Sabatin Bascoban, Sandra Faidi, Guadalupe Méndez Cárdenas, Katrin Heimberger, and Mal-Hie Im for their love, moral support, encouragement, and patience.

GENERAL REFERENCES

Aitken, M. L., Franklin, J. L., Pierson, D. J., & Schoene, R. B. 1986 Influence of body size and gender on control of ventilation. J. Appl. Physiol. 60, 1894-1899.

Anderson, J.R., Myowa-Yamakoshi, M., & Matsuzawa, T. 2004 Contagious yawning in chimpanzees. Proc. R. Soc. B 271, 468-470.

Archangelsky, M. 2004 Higher-level phylogeny of Hydrophilinae (Coleoptera: Hydrophilidae) based on larval, pupal and adult characters. Syst. Entomol. 29, 188-214.

Bachorowski, J.-A. & Owren, M.J. 2001 Not all laughs are alike: Voiced but not unvoiced laughter readily elicits positive affect. Psych. Science 12 (3), 252-257.

Bachorowski, J.-A., Smoski, M.J., & Owren, M.J. 2001 The acoustic features of human laughter. J. Acoust. Soc. Am. 110, 1581-1597.

Baldwin, J.D. & Baldwin, J.I. 1976 Vocalizations of howler monkeys (*Alouatta palliata*) in Southwestern Panama. Folia Primatol. 26, 81-108.

Bard, K. 2006 Neonatal imitation in chimpanzees (*Pan troglodytes*) tested with two paradigms. Anim. Cogn.

Bekoff, M. & Byers, J.A. 1981 A critical reanalysis of the ontogeny and phylogeny of mammalian social and locomotor play: an ethological hornet's nest. In Behavioral development (eds. K. Immelmann, G. Barlow, M. Main, & L. Petrinovich), pp. 296-337. Cambridge: Cambridge University Press.

Bekoff, M. 1995 Play signals as punctuation: The structure of social play in canids. Behaviour 132 (5-6), 419-429.

Bekoff, M. 1999 Social cognition: Exchanging and sharing information on the run. Erkenntnis 51, 113–128.

Berntson, G.G., Boysen, S.T., Bauer, H.R., & Torello M.S. 1989 Conspecific screams and laughter: Cardiac and behavioral reactions of infant chimpanzees. Dev. Psychobiol. 22 (8), 771-787.

Biben, M. 1998 Squirrel monkey play fighting: making the case for a cognitive training function for play. In Animal play: Evolutionary, comparative, and ecological perspectives (eds. M. Bekoff & J.A. Byers), pp. 161-182. Cambridge: Cambridge University Press.

Blurton Jones, N.G. 1967 An ethological study of some aspects of social behaviour of children in nursery school. In Primate ethology (ed. D. Morris). pp 347–368. London: Weidenfeld and Nicolson.

Boersma, P. & Weenink, D. 2007. Praat: Doing phonetics by computer (Version 4.5.16) [Computer program]. Retrieved February 18.

Braune,P. 2006 Acoustic variability and its biological significance in noctural lemurs, Hannover: Universität Hannover, 100 p.

Caron, J.E. 2002 From ethology to aesthetics: Evolution as a theoretical paradigm for research on laughter, humor, and other comic phenomena. Humor 15 (3), 245-281.

Chevalier-Skolnikoff, S. 1982 A cognitive analysis of facial behavior in Old World monkeys, apes, and human beings. Primate communication, (eds. C.T. Snowdon, C.H. Brown, & M.R. Petersen), pp. 303-368. Cambridge: Cambridge University Press.

Cleveland, J. & Snowdon, C.T. 1982 The complex vocal repertoire of the adult cotton-top tamarin (*Saguinus oedipus oedipus*). Z. Tierpsychol. 58, 231-270.

Davila Ross, M. & Geissmann, T. 2007 Call diversity of wild male orangutans: A phylogenetic approach. Am. J. Primatol. 69, 305-324.

de Waal, F.B.M. 1988 The communicative repertoire of captive bonobos (*Pan paniscus*) compared to that of chimpanzees. Behaviour 106, 183-251.

de Waal, F.B.M. 1995 Bonobo sex ans society: the behavior of a close relative challenges assumptions about male supremacy in human evolution. Sci. Am. 272, 82-88.

de Waal, F.B.M. 2001 Apes from Venus: bonobos and human social evolution. Tree of origin: What primate behavior can tell us about human social evolution (ed. F.B.M. de Waal), p. 41-68. Cambridge: Harvard University Press.

Decety, J. & Jackson, P.L. 2006 A social-neuroscience perspective on empathy. Curr. Direct. Psychol. Sci. 15 (2), 54–58.

Delgado, R.A. & van Schaik, C.P. 2000. The behavioral ecology and conservation of the orangutan (*Pongo pygmaeus*). A tale of two islands. Evol. Anthrop. 9:201-218.

Dimberg, U. & Thunberg, M. 1998 Rapid facial reactions to emotional facial expressions. Scand. J. of Psychol. 39, 39-45.

Dimberg, U., Thunberg, M. & Elmehed, K. 2000 Unconscious facial reactions to emotional facial expressions. Psychol. Sci. 11, 86-89.

Eibl-Eibesfeldt, I. 1985 Der vorprogrammierte Mensch. Kiel: Orion-Heimreiter-Verlag.

Ekman, P. 1973 Cross-cultural studies of facial expression. In Darwin and Facial Expression (ed. P. Ekman), pp. 169–222. New York: Academic Press.

Ekman, P. 2003 Emotions Revealed: Recognizing faces and feelings to improve communication and emotional life. New York: Times Books

Eriksson, E.J., Cepeda, L.F., Rodman, R.D., McAlister, D.F., Bitzer, D., & Arroway, P. 2004 Cross-language speaker identification using spectral moments. Fonetik, Dept. of Linguistics, Stockholm University.

Fagan, R.M. 1981 Animal play behavior. New York: Oxford University Press.

Farris, J. 1989. The retention index and the resealed consistency index. Cladistics 5, 417-419.

Felsenstein, J. 1985 Confidence limits on phylogenies: An approach using the bootstrap. Evolution 39 (4), 783-791.

Ferrari, P.F., Gallese, V., Rizzolatti, G., & Fogassi, L. 2003 Mirror neurons responding to the observation of ingestive and communicative mouth actions in the monkey ventral premotor cortex. Eur. J. Neurosci. 17 (8), 1703–1714.

Ferrari, P.F., Visalberghi, E., Paukner, A., Fogassi, L., Ruggiero, A., Suomi, S.J. 2006 Neonatal imitation in rhesus macaques. PLoS Biol. 4(9), e302.

Fischer, J., Hammerschmidt, K., Cheney, D.L., Seyfarth, R.M. 2001 Acoustic features of female chacma baboon barks. Ethology 107(1), 33-54.

Fitch, W.T. 2000 The evolution of speech: a comparative review. Trends Cognit. Sci. 4, 258-267.

Fitch, W.T., Neubauer, J., & Herzel, H. 2002 Calls out of chaos: the adaptive significance of nonlinear phenomena in mammalian vocal production. Anim. Behav. 63, 407-418.

Flack, J.C., Jeannotte, L.A., & de Waal, F.B.M. 2004 Play signaling and the perception of social rules by juvenile chimpanzees (Pan troglodytes). J. Comp. Psychol. 118, 149-159.

Fleiss, J.L., Levin, B., & Paik, M.C. 2003 Statistical methods for rates and proportions, 3rd edn. New York: John Wiley & Sons.

Förderreuther, B. & Zimmermann, E. 2003 "Laughter" in bonobos?: Preliminary results of an acoustic analysis of tickling sounds in a hand-reared male. Folia Primatol. 74, 193-194.

Fossey, D. 1983 Gorillas in the mist. Boston: Houghton Mifflin.

Freedman, J.L. & Perlick, D. 1979 Crowding, contagion, and laughter. J. Exp. Soc. Psychol. 15, 295-303.

Garcia-Cruz, J. & Sosa, V. 2006 Coding quantitative character data for phylogenetic analysis: A comparison of five methods. Syst. Botany 31(2), 302-309.

Geissmann, T. 1984 Inheritance of song parameters in the gibbon song, analysed in 2 hybrid gibbons (*Hylobates pileatus* x *H. lar*). Folia Primatol. 42, 216-235.

Gervais, M., Wilson, D.S. 2005 The evolution and functions of laughter and humor: a synthetic approach. Quart. Rev. Biol. 80, 395-430.

Goodall, J. 1986 The chimpanzees of Gombe: Patterns of behavior. Cambridge: Harvard University Press.

Goodman, M., Porter, C.A., Czelusniak, J., Page, S.L., Schneider, H., Shoshani, J., Gunnell, G., & Groves, C.P. 1998 Towards a phylogenetic classification of primates based on DNA evidence complemented by fossil evidence. Mol. Phylogenet. Evol. 9, 585-598.

Grammer, K. & Eibl-Eibesfeldt, I. 1990 The ritualisation of laughter. In: Natürlichkeit der Sprache und der Kultur (ed. W.A. Koch) pp 192-214. Bochum: Universitätsverlag, Dr. Norbert Brockmeyer.

Harris, C. 1999 The mystery of ticklish laughter. American Scientist 87(4), 344-350.

Hatfield, E., Cacioppo, J.T. & Rapson, R.L. 1994 Emotional contagion, Cambridge: Cambridge University Press.

Hess, U. & Blairy, S. 2001 Facial mimicry and emotional contagion to dynamic emotional facial expressions and their influence on decoding accuracy. Int. J. Psychophysiol. 40, 129-141.

Hochberg, Y. & Hommel, G. 1998 Step-up multiple testing procedures. Encyclopedia Statist. Sci. (Supp.) 2.

Jenkins, P.A. 1987 Catalogue of primates in the British Museum (Natural History) and elsewhere in the British Isles. Part 4: Suborder Strepsirrhini, including the subfossil Madagascaran lemurs and family Tarsiidae. London: British Museum.

Jürgens, U. 2002a A study of the central control of vocalization using the squirrel monkey. Med. Eng. Phys. 24, 473-477.

Jürgens, U. 2002b Neural pathways underlying vocal control. Neurosci. Biobehav. Rev. 26, 235-258.

Kipper, S. & Todt, D. 2001 Variation of sound parameters affects the evaluation of human laughter. Behaviour 138, 1161-1178.

Kitching, I.J., Forey, P.L., Humphries, C.J., & Williams, D.M. 1998 Cladistics: The theory and practice of parsimony analysis. New York: Oxford University Press. xiii+228 p.

Kojima, S. 2001 Early vocal development in a chimpanzee infant. Primate origins of human cognition and behavior (ed. T. Matsuzawa), pp. 190-196. Tokyo: Springer-Verlag.

Ladygina-Kohts, N.N. 1935/2002 Infant chimpanzee and human child: A classic 1935 comparative study of ape emotions and intelligence (ed. F.B.M. de Waal) New York: Oxford University Press.

Lieberman, P. 1975 On the origins of language: An introduction to the evolution of human speech. New York: Macmillan.

Lieberman, P., Klatt, D. H., & Wilson, W. H. 1969 Vocal tract limitations on the vowel repertoires of rhesus monkeys and other nonhuman primates. Science 164, 1185-1187.

Lieberman, D.E. 1984 The biology and evolution of language. Cambridge: Harvard University Press.

Lieberman, D.E., McCarthy, R.C., Hiiemae, K.M. & Palmer, J.B. 2001 Ontogeny of postnatal hyoid and larynx descent in humans. Arch. Oral Biol. 46, 117-128.

Locke, J.L., Bekken, K.E., McMinn-Larson, L. & Wein, D. 1995 Emergent control of manual and vocal-motor activity in relation to the development of speech. Brain Lang. 51, 498-508.

Lundqvist, L.-O. 1995 Facial EMG reactions to facial expressions: A case of facial emotional contagion? Scand. J. of Psychol. 36, 130-141.

Macedonia J.M. & Stanger K.F. 1994. Phylogeny of the Lemuridae revisited: Evidence from communication signals. Folia Primatol. 63, 1-43.

MacLarnon, A. & Hewitt, G. 2004 Increased breathing control: another factor in the evolution of human language. Evol. Anthropol. 13:181-197.

MacLarnon, A.M. & Hewitt, G.P. 1999 The evolution of human speech: the role of enhanced breathing control. Am. J. Phys. Anthropol. 109:341-363.

Maddison, D.R. & Maddison, W.P. 2000. MacClade 4: Analysis of phylogeny and character evolution. Sunderland, Massachusetts: Sinauer Associates. 492 p.

Marler, P. & Tenaza, R. 1977 Signaling behavior of apes with special reference to vocalization. How animals communicate (ed. T. A. Seboek) pp. 965-1033, Bloomington: Indiana University Press.

Marler, P. 1976 Social organization, communication and graded signals: the chimpanzee and the gorilla. Growing points in ethology. (ed. Hinde, R.A.) pp. 239-280, Cambridge: Cambridge Univ Press.

Marshall, A.J., Wrangham, R.W., & Arcadi, A.C. 1999. Does learning affect the structure of vocalizations in chimpanzees? Anim. Behav. 58, 825-830.

Matsusaka, T. 2004 When does play panting occur during social play in wild chimpanzees? Primates 45, 221-229.

McBrearty,S. & Jablonski, N.G. First fossil chimpamzee. Nature 437 (1.9.), 105-108, 2005.

Meltzoff, A.N. & Moore, M.K. 1997 Explaining facial imitation: A theoretical model. Early Dev. Parenting 6, 179-192.

Mitani, J.C. 1996 Comparative studies of African ape vocal behavior. Great ape societies. (eds W.C McGrew & L.F. Marchant & T. Nishida) pp. 241-254. Cambridge: Cambridge University Press.

Mori, A. 1984 An ethological study of pygmy chimpanuees in Wambs, Zaire: a comparison with chimpanzees. Primates 25, 255-278.

Myowa-Yamakoshi, M., Tomonaga, M., Tanaka, M., & Matsuzawa, T. 2004 Imitation in neonatal chimpanzees (*Pan troglodytes*). Dev. Sci. 7(4), 437-442

Newman, J.D. & Symmes, D. 1982 Inheritance and experience in the acquisition of primate acoustic behavior. Primate communication (ed. C.T. Snowdon, C.H. Brown, & M.R. Petersen) pp.259-278. Cambridge: Cambridge University Press.

Nishimura, T., Mikami, A., Suzuki, J., & Matsuzawa, T. 2003 Descent of the larynx in chimpanzee infants. Proc. Natl. Acad. Sci. U.S.A. 100 (12):6930-6933.

Nwokah, E.E., Davies, P., Islam, A. 1993 Vocal affect in three-year-olds: A quantitative acoustic analysis of child laughter. J. Acoust. Soc. Am. 94, 3076-3090.

Owren, M.J., Seyfarth, R.M., & Cheney, D.L. 1997. The acoustic features of vowel-like grunt calls in chacma baboons (*Papio cynocephalus ursinus*): Implications for production processes and functions. J. Acoust. Soc. Am., 101, 2951-2963.

Panksepp, J. & Burgdorf, J. 2003 "Laughing" rats and the evolutionary antecedents of human joy? Physiol. Behav. 79, 533-547.

Parr, L.A. 2001 Cognitive and physiological markers of emotional awareness in chimpanzees (*Pan troglodytes*). Anim. Cogn. 4, 223-229.

Patterson, C. 1988 Homology in classical and molecular biology. Mol. Biol. Evol. 5(6), 603-625.

Paukner, A. & Anderson, J.R. 2006 Video-induced yawning in stumptail macaques (*Macaca arctoides*). Biol. Lett. 2, 36-38.

Platek, S.M., Critton, S.R., Myers, T.E. & Gallup G.G. 2003 Contagious yawning: the role of self-awareness and mental state attribution. Cogn. Brain Res. 17, 223-227.

Preston, S.D. & de Waal, F.B.M. 2002 Empathy: Its ultimate and proximate bases. Behav. Brain Sci. 25, 1-72.

Preuschoft, S. 1995 'Laughter' and 'smiling' in macaques - an evolutionary perspective. Utrecht: Rijksuniversiteit, 254 p.

Provine, R.R. 1992 Contagious laughter: laughter is a sufficient stimulus for laughs and smiles. Bull. Psychonom. Soc. 30 (1), 1-4.

Provine, R.R. 1993 Laughter punctuates speech: linguistic, social and gender contexts of laughter. Ethology 95, 291-298.

Provine, R.R. 1996 Laughter. Am. Sci. 84, 38-45.

Provine, R.R. 2000 Laughter: a scientific investigation, New York: Penguin Books.

Provine, R.R. 2004 Laughing, tickling, and the evolution of speech and self. Curr. Direct. Psychol. Sci. 13 (6), 215-218.

Redican, W.K. 1982 An evolutionary perspective on human facial displays. Emotion in the human face (ed. P. Ekman), p. 212-281. Cambridge: Cambridge University Press.

Riede, T., Owren, M.J., & Arcadi, A.C. 2004 Nonlinear acoustics in pant hoots of common chimpanzees (*Pan troglodytes*): Frequency jumps, subharmonics, biphonation, and deterministic chaos. Am. J. Primatol. 64, 277–291.

Riedo, T., Wilden, I., & Tembrock, G. 1997 Subharmonics, biphonations, and frequency jumps - common components of mammalian vocalization or indicators for disorders? Z Säugetier 62 (Suppl 2):198–203.

Rijksen, H.D. 1978. A fieldstudy on Sumatran orang utans (*Pongo pygmaeus abelii*, Lesson 1827). Ecology, behaviour and conservation. Wageningen: Veenman H, Zones BV.

Robillard, T., Höbel, G. & Gerhardt, H.C. 2006 Evolution of advertising signals in North American hylid frogs: Vocalizations as end-products of calling behavior. Cladistics 22, 1-13.

Robins, R.L. & McCreery, E.K. 2003 African wild dog pup vocalizations with special reference to Morton's Model. Behaviour 140, 333-351.

Rodman, R., McAllister, D., Bitzer, D. Cepeda, L., & Abbit, P. 2002 Forensic speaker identification based on spectral moments. Forensic Linguistics 9(1), 1350-1771.

Rothbart, M.K. 1973 Laughter in young children. Psych. Bull. 80, 247-256.

Rothgänger, H., Hauser, G., Cappelini, A.C., & Guidotti, A. 1998 Analysis of laughter and speech sounds in Italian and German students. Naturwissenschaften 85, 394-402.

Rowe, N. 1996 The pictorial guide to the living primates. East Hampton, New York: Pogonias Press.

Ruch, W. & Ekman, P. 2001 The expressive pattern of laughter. Emotion, qualia and consciousness (ed A. Kazniak) pp. 426-443.Tokyo: World Scientifc.

Ruvolo, M., Pan, D., Zehr, S., Goldberg, T., Disotell, T.R. & von Dornum, M. 1994 Gene trees and hominoid phylogeny. Proc. Natl. Acad. Sci. USA. 91, 8900-8904.

Scheiner, E., Hammerschmidt, K., Jürgens, U. & Zwirner, P. 2002 Acoustic analyses of developmental changes and emotional expression in the preverbal vocalizations of infants. J. Voice 16 (4), 509-529.

Schenkel, R. 1964 Zur Ontogenese des Verhaltens bei Gorilla und Mensch. Zeitschrift Morphologie und Anthropologie. 54, 233-259

Siegel, S. 1956 Nonparametric statistics for the behavioral sciences, 1st edn. New York: McGraw-Hill Book Company.

Smoski, M.J. & Bachorowski, J.-A. 2003 Antiphonal laughter between friends and strangers. Cogn. Emotion 17, 327-340.

Sroufe, L.A. & Wunsch, J.P. 1972 The development of laughter in the first year of life. Child Devel. 43,1326-1344.

Stevenson, M.F. & Poole, T.B. 1982 Playful interactions in family groups of the common marmoset (*Callithrix jacchus jacchus*). Anim. Behav. 30, 886-900.

Struhsaker, T.T. 1975 The red colobus monkey. Chicago: University of Chicago Press.

Swofford, D.L. 1990, PAUP: Phylogenetic analysis using parsimony. Campaign, Illinois: Computer program distributed by Illinois Natural History Survey (3).

Tabachnick, B.G. & Fidell, L.S. 2007 *Using multivariate statistics*, Boston: Pearson Education, Inc.

Taglialatela, J.P., Savage-Rumbaugh, E.S., & Baker, L.A. 2003 Vocal production by a language competent *Pan paniscus*. Int. J. Primatol. 24 (1).

Thiele, K. 1993 The holy grail of the perfect character: The cladistic treatment of morphometric data. Cladistics 9, 275-304.

Tokuda, I., Riede,T., Neubauer, J., Owren, M.J., & Herzel, H-P. 2002 Nonlinear analysis of irregular animal vocalizations. J. Acoust. Soc. Am. 111, 2908-2919.

van Hooff, J.A.R.A.M. & Preuschoft, S. 2003 Laughter and Smiling: the intertwining of nature and culture. In Animal Social Complexity: Intelligence, culture, and individualized societies (eds F.B.M. de Waal & P.L. Tyack), pp 261-287. Cambridge: Harvard University Press.

van Hooff, J.A.R.A.M. 1967 The facial displays of the Catarrhine monkeys and apes. In Primate Ethology (ed. D. Morris), pp. 7-68. London: Weidenfeld and Nicholson.

van Hooff, J.A.R.A.M. 1972 A comparative approach to the phylogeny of laughter and smiling. Non-verbal communication (ed. R. A. Hinde), pp. 209-241. Cambridge: Cambridge University Press.

van Schaik, C.P. 1999 The socioecology of fission–fusion sociality in orangutans. Primates 40, 73-90.

Vettin, J. & Todt, D. 2004 Laughter in conversation: Features of occurrence and acoustic structure. J. Nonverb. Behav. 28 (2), 93-115.

Vettin, J. & Todt, D. 2005 Human laughter, social play, and play vocalizations of non-human primates: an evolutionary approach. Behaviour 142, 217-240.

Waller, B.M. & Dunbar, R.I.M. 2005 Differential behavioural effects of silent bared teeth display and relaxed open mouth display in chimpanzees (Pan troglodytes). Ethology 111, 129-142.

Watts, D.P. & Pusey, A.E. 1993 Behavior of juvenile and adolescent great apes. In Juvenile Primates: Life History, Development, and Behavior (eds. M.E. Pereira & L.A. Fairbanks), pp. 148-172. New York: Oxford University Press.

Weisfeld, G.E. 1993 The adaptive value of humor and laughter. Ethol. Sociobiol. 14, 141-169.

Wild, B., Erb, M., Eyb, M., Bartels, M. & Grodd, W. 2003 Why are smiles contagious? An fMRI study of the interaction between perception of facial affect and facial movements. Psychiatry Res. 123, 17-36.

Wildman, D.E., Grossman, L.I., & Goodman, M. 2002 Functional DNA in humans and chimpanzees shows that they are more similar to each other than either is to other apes. Probing human origins (eds. M. Goodman, A.S. Moffat), pp. 1-10. Cambridge: American Academy of Arts and Sciences.

Winkworth, A.L., Davis, P.J., Adams, [2] R.D., Ellis, E. 1995 Breathing patterns during spontaneous speech. J. Speech Hear. Res. 38. 124-144.

Zimmermann, E. 1989 Aspects of reproduction and behavioral and vocal development in Senegal bushbabies (Galago senegalensis). Int. J. Primatol. 10 (1), 1-17.

Zimmermann, E. 1990 Differentiation of vocalizations in bushbabies (Galaginae, Prosimiae, Primates) and the significance for assessing phylogenetic relationships. Z Zool Syst Evol-forschg 28, 217-239.

Zimmermann, E. 1991 Ontogeny of acoustic communication in prosimian primates. Primatology today (eds. A. Ehara, O. Takenaka, & M. Iwamoto), pp. 337-340. Amsterdam: Elsevier.

Zimmermann, E. 1995 Loud calls in nocturnal prosimians: structure, evolution and ontogeny. Current topics in primate vocal communication (eds. E. Zimmermann, J. D. Newman, & U. Jürgens) p. 47-72, New York: Plenum Press.

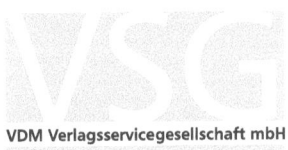

Die VDM Verlagsservicegesellschaft sucht für wissenschaftliche Verlage abgeschlossene und herausragende

Dissertationen, Habilitationen, Diplomarbeiten, Master Theses, Magisterarbeiten usw.

für die kostenlose Publikation als Fachbuch.

Sie verfügen über eine Arbeit, die hohen inhaltlichen und formalen Ansprüchen genügt, und haben Interesse an einer honorarvergüteten Publikation?

Dann senden Sie bitte erste Informationen über sich und Ihre Arbeit per Email an *info@vdm-vsg.de*.

Sie erhalten kurzfristig unser Feedback!

VDM Verlagsservicegesellschaft mbH
Dudweiler Landstr. 99
D - 66123 Saarbrücken
www.vdm-vsg.de

Telefon +49 681 3720 174
Fax   +49 681 3720 1749

Die VDM Verlagsservicegesellschaft mbH vertritt

 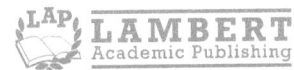 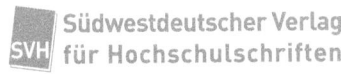

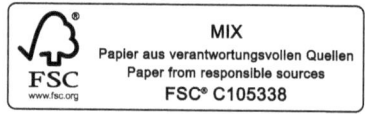

Printed by Books on Demand GmbH, Norderstedt / Germany